MW01235699

My Wife Has Cancer

A Story of Love, Relationship, & The One Left Behind

By Rocco Ciaramella

authorHOUSE™

1663 LIBERTY DRIVE, SUITE 200
BLOOMINGTON, INDIANA 47403
(800) 839-8640
WWW.AUTHORHOUSE.COM

First published by AuthorHouse 05/19/05

ISBN: 1-4208-1511-3 (sc)
ISBN: 1-4208-1512-1 (dj)

Printed in the United States of America
Bloomington, Indiana

This book is printed on acid-free paper.

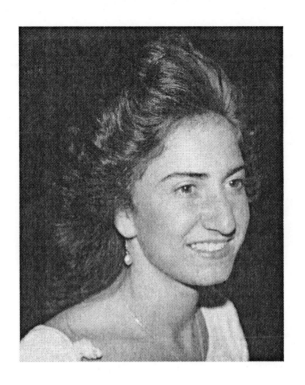

Annette Ciaramella

I dedicate this book in memory
of my loving wife, Annette
Ciaramella.

Her faith and spirit brought joy
to the lives of everyone she met.

Until the day that we are
reunited, know that my love
for you is an eternal flame that
lights up my soul.

Table of Contents

Foreword

Foreword

I started writing this book as a means of unloading all of the emotion and anxiety that came with taking care of Annette. Cancer is a horrifying disease that doesn't recognize age, color of skin, ethnic background, financial status, or whether you're a good person or not. It doesn't care who gets left behind in the wake. It attacks babies, small children, and single parents with kids at home that rely on them for the basic essentials of life. It will snatch a life with the same disregard, whether you are a war hero or a convicted child molester.

Originally, this started as a journal, a diary of sorts that contained a myriad of ideas and thoughts . . . the pages filled with unguided emotion, packed with despair and anger that rambled on, going off in many different directions. Yes, it was a place to unload, but it wasn't bringing any peace. I would write without any focal point. Encouraged by Annette, I changed focus and began to structure it not so much as a guide but as a testimony to what we endured and how it affected everything that we treasured. This new focus forced me to come to terms with what was happening. It gave me the courage to go forward and live. This demon took Annette's life; I WILL NOT allow it to also destroy my life or our boy's lives.

First and foremost, this book is for the spouses. I would like to think it helps those who have experienced the pain firsthand to know they are not alone. (Please note, I didn't say comfort them in their loss. As you read on, you will find that knowing someone else has experienced the pain will not, nor should it, bring any comfort to you.) This book is to let you know that you are not alone; there are thousands of us walking the streets and working through our daily lives one step at a time. What you have to understand is that whatever you are experiencing is unique to your relationship between you and the one you love. No one can tell you how long it will take you to return to a "normal" life or how long it takes you to be able to look at a picture or hear a song without curling up in a ball, sobbing yourself to sleep. Don't be surprised if you find yourself standing in the middle of the grocery store crying because you just passed your spouse's favorite food. Every one of us has walked the unbeaten path that was laid before us. That trail will pass through the dark forest of anguish and pain, and you will stumble and fall just as a baby does when they take those first steps. All I can tell you is keep going, keep fighting. There is light at the end of the forest. Don't let that demon take any more lives than it already has. Reach out for help; there is an army of people ready and willing to help you along. Please don't be afraid or too proud to ask.

I also wrote this book for the close family members and friends with the hopes that it provides some insight into how tragic the loss of a spouse can be, especially at such a young age.

It is my wish that our experience and my thoughts shed some light on and bring awareness to the importance of supporting such organizations as

American Cancer Society
St. Jude Children's Research Hospital
and
The Hospice program.

In support of those organizations, a portion of the proceeds from the sale of this book will be donated in memory of my wife Annette.

With your help and support and the grace of God, one day these brilliant people will find a way to conquer the oppressor, bringing hope and peace to all who face the uncertainty of this debilitating disease.

Chapter 1

In the Beginning

November 2, 2002, was a Saturday, and we had friends coming over for dinner. As usual, I worked a half a day, and when I came home, Annette was busy cleaning and getting things ready. We live in what I guess would be considered a suburb of Detroit. Twenty-five years ago people bought property out here and built vacation cottages. Well, with the expansion of industry along the I-75 corridor, modern suburbia has stretched its way up to and past the boundaries of our small town of Lake Orion.

Our love nest is what is known as a tri-level home. There is no basement, and the levels are staggered, with four steps down to the lower level and six steps that take you from the middle level to the upper level. Over the last seven years we have completely remodeled our modest home to reflect your average suburban home with a hint of lakefront cottage. The living room is sunken in one step from the rest of the middle level. On the back wall above the leather furniture you will find Annette's lighthouse collection that I mounted on real pieces of slate. Over in the dining room you will find her magnet collection tastefully displayed on two separate tri-fold picture frames. A ceramic tile floor greets you at the foyer and continues on into the kitchen that we just completely remodeled. As you walk in the front door, there hangs a plaque that reads, " *A fisherman lives here and so does the best catch of his life.* Today I cherish that plaque as a memorial to everything Annette and I shared.

Anyway, I found Annette in the kitchen standing at the sink. When I walked in from the garage, she turned to see who came in, and just as she always did, she said, "Hi, honey," accompanied by an alluring smile. Seeing her arms buried up to her elbows in dishwater, I came up from behind, wrapped my arms around her, and kissed the soft nape of her neck. I rested my chin on her shoulder and asked where the boys were. She replied they were outside playing football with their friends. That answer was worth a few more kisses and a little more caressing. It never seemed

1

to take much for us to get going. You would never guess we were married for almost twenty years the way we carried on when given the slightest opportunity.

Our guests Tom and Sally arrived around six that evening. Sally worked with Annette a few years back at one of the local companies. As with most of our friends the relationship started With Annette. It's not that I'm anti social, I just don't get that close to other people as quickly as Annette does. Like any other dinner party we sat around and socialized as the meal finished cooking. The night was going as scheduled, we ate dinner, had dessert, and were exchanging stories in the living room when, all of a sudden, Annette was not feeling well; in fact, she felt so bad that our company went home early.

It was the strangest thing—everything was so normal one minute, and the next, excruciating pain.

As I said before, she spent the day cleaning and cooking in preparation for an evening with friends. We enjoyed a wonderful meal and were relaxing on the couch, when all of a sudden, just as if someone hit her with a baseball bat, Annette was in pain.

We saw this couple maybe two times a year, and when we did get together, it was easily a twelve-to-one-o'clock-in-the-morning kind of visit. Yet, on this particular evening, our friends said good night at eight o'clock.

Annette's pain was so bad that for the next two nights she slept sitting up with a pillow on her lap. I know what you are thinking: why did she wait two days before going to the doctor? All I can say is you have to know Annette; she doesn't like doctors' offices or taking medicine and will avoid them the way a fish avoids dry land.

I've told that scenario to probably a hundred people by now, everyone from family and friends to a countless number of doctors and nurses that needed to know how this all began.

This kind of thing shouldn't be happening to her. Annette exercised every day, watched what she ate, and stayed very active. She's not supposed to get ill—not like this.

If anyone in our family is a candidate, it is me. I should be the one sick, not Annette. I only exercise when she forces me to, I rarely eat a well-balanced diet, and I work too long and don't sleep enough. This should not be happening to my wife.

I just don't understand! Why is this happening to Annette?

Today is the seventeenth of January 2003. It has been a little over ten weeks since Annette first felt the pain. I told her the other day that I was going to write a book about what has happened to us. She was all for it. She knows I won't go see anyone or talk about what I'm going through, so this gives me a way to unload some of the things that I'm feeling.

When you read this book, you have to keep in mind that there hasn't been any research; the only facts that you can count on is how this horrid disease has affected her life, my life, and the lives of our three boys. I'm not saying that what has happened to us will happen to you or that you should do the things we have done because they worked for us. All I'm doing is putting down on paper my thoughts as this thing unfolds.

If for some reason you find correlation between your experience and ours, then take comfort in knowing that you are not alone and there is always hope. **What . . . A . . . Crock!** that last statement is. There is no comfort. People that say things like that have not experienced the pain.

I challenge you to gather one thousand people who have struggled through a debilitating disease or lost a loved one to it. Then ask them if there is any comfort knowing that others also lost someone they loved. Do you know what they are going to say? They're going to say **NO!**

The loss of a loved one, or a spouse, cannot be comforted by knowing someone else has suffered.

Just for a moment, imagine there are two ladies, two mothers, walking down the street. Both have just recently learned that their son or daughter was killed overseas fighting the war on terrorism, and they are overwhelmed with grief. They begin a conversation in which they exchange memories of their children and show each other pictures of their children that were taken not so long ago. Maybe they are graduation pictures from high school or maybe they are family photos that include a wife or husband along with their children at ages one, three and six. Now imagine at the end of the conversation their grief and horror is comforted. **YEAH, RIGHT!**

You can feel sympathy, you may even be able to understand the other's misery, but it will not comfort the loss. Only someone who hasn't felt the agony would make a idiotic statement like that. Does it help to talk to others that have experienced a similar tragedy? I'm sure it does, but it won't remove the pain. I have talked to other people, and they tell me that the pain never really goes away. If you are lucky, you're able to put it away. It's not forgotten, but it's in a place that allows you to carry on and enjoy this wonderful world.

I've never written a book before; in fact, I haven't read many either. I prefer articles. I just don't seem to have the time to read a novel. This book is more like a consolidation of thoughts than it is about a story. Stories have plots and endings and, as of now, we don't know how this is going to end. Cancer isn't about plots and themes; it is about many different aspects of your life that are brought to the forefront, and none of them have anything to do with the other except for the fact that, as of this moment, you have to deal with all of them and not necessarily one at a time.

The Journey

November 2, 8:00 p.m. —The pain hits. I was sitting in the recliner, Tom was on the loveseat, and Sally was sitting next to Annette on the couch. I began to notice that Annette wasn't participating in the conversation like she normally did. Her face began to flinch from the pain.

I asked her, "What's wrong, honey?"

"I have a pain in my side, but I'll be alright," Annette said.

I let it go for a little while. Then I noticed that she had slid down on the couch, kind of half laying and half sitting.

"Are you sure you're alright?" I asked. "You don't look too good."

"It really hurts," she replied. "All of a sudden I started feeling this pain in my side."

"Do you feel nauseous?" I asked.

"No," she said.

Then we all agreed it couldn't have been the food, because we all ate the same thing, and the rest of us were feeling fine. Annette then said she thought it felt like she had pulled a muscle or bruised a rib.

About three weeks earlier she had moved some boxes in the car that were too heavy for her, and she pulled or strained a muscle in her shoulder. We thought maybe this had something to do with that. Maybe she aggravated her rib, and it was rebelling. Annette was in a lot of pain, so Sally and Tom decided to go home. As I stated before, the pain was so bad Annette had to sleep sitting up with a pillow on her lap. Thinking she bruised a rib, she spends two days in bed before going to the doctor.

It was Tuesday, November 5th. Two days have passed since the pain had begun. I left for work early like I always do. It's a forty-mile commute to the shop, so I leave around five thirty to beat rush-hour traffic. I woke our eldest son, Nick, and told him that Mom was still sick and to spread the word to his brothers that I didn't want a bunch of commotion this morning. "Just get up and do what you have to do to get ready for school."

Normally, Annette would get up, make breakfast, and spend some quiet time with them. Well, I don't know about the quiet time—we're talking about three boys aged nine to thirteen. If you have kids, you know

5

what I'm talking about. Ever since they were in kindergarten, we left it to them to make their own lunch and collect what they needed for school the next day. We supervised them, but it was their responsibility to get everything together. With our youngest now in fourth grade, they're used to getting their things together and getting off to school, so I wasn't very concerned about leaving and letting them fend for themselves.

Later that morning Annette called me at work and told me that the pain wasn't getting any better, so she made an appointment to go see our family doctor, Dr. William Brewer. Around eleven thirty, I received a call from her: "Bill (Dr. Brewer) is sending me to the emergency room at the hospital. He thinks I'm having a severe gallbladder attack."

"OK," I said. "I'll meet you there."

From the shop to the hospital is about a forty-five-minute drive. Bill's office is ten minutes away. When I finally made it to the emergency room, I went straight back to the beds. We spend a lot of time in the emergency room. If it's not the boys getting repaired, it's me. So we're familiar with the workings of the emergency room.

I have to stop and tell you this story before I go any further. When Annette and I moved back from Las Vegas to Michigan, we bought a small house in Auburn Hills. It was a small 980-square-foot three-bedroom ranch. Well, with our third son Jacob on the way, we set up a full-size bed in one bedroom that Nick and Zack shared to make room in the nursery for Jacob. At the time Nick was four and Zack was around two and a half years old. One evening they were wrestling around in the bedroom, so I told them to settle down and go to sleep. As kids do, they ignored me, so I called them out to the family room, so I could tell them sternly that I wanted them to go to sleep. Right, as much as you want to think that, as a parent, you are the supreme commander, your kids are the ones that are in control. The best you can do is to find a way to outthink them. Anyway, while they are standing in front of me, and I'm giving out my directive to cease and desist, Nick informs me that Zack was sticking a Peg Light bulb up his nose. So I turn to Zack and demand that he stop this and get to sleep.

Nick yells, "No, Dad!! "He stuck a Peg Yite bulb up my nose."

6

Keep in mind I'm talking to a four-year-old.

"What do you mean he stuck a Peg Light bulb up your nose," I asked.

"Look," he said, as he tilted his head back.

At this point I could see Annette sitting on the couch trying to hold back her laughter. I went and got the flashlight and, sure enough, there was a red plastic Peg Light bulb buried deep in his nasal cavity.

With a look of disbelief on my face, I asked "Nick, why did you let him do that?"

"I didn't," he cries out. "I was sleeping."

I turned to Zack, and he was standing there with this big smile on his face. Zack's smile is irresistible. He has a humor about him that just fills the room. I looked at Annette, and she was losing it. I couldn't help but start laughing. While I was getting Nick dressed I told Annette to call the emergency room and let them know we were on our way. It was ten o'clock at night, and I was on my way to the hospital with Nick to have this bulb removed. Poor Nick, he was the only one that night that didn't see the humor in it.

Getting back to the story. As I said, Annette was much closer to the hospital than I was, and I thought for sure she would have been admitted and receiving treatment by the time I made arrangements at work and drove to the hospital. Our hospital is not very big or busy; you usually can walk right in and get treated. When I couldn't find her, I went to the nurses' station and asked if they had taken her anywhere. With her having this gallbladder attack I thought maybe they took her right to surgery. The nurse informs me that she hasn't been admitted yet and that I should check at the registration desk. This is where I find her. Looking around I could see they weren't busy, there was only one other person in the waiting room, and he had a pile of coats with him, so I figured he came with someone, and they were already in being treated.

So I asked, "What took you so long to get here?"

To my disbelief, she tells me that before coming to the hospital she stopped to pick up some things that she had her mother buy at the store for us.

I couldn't believe it. She could hardly walk, Bill tells her to go to the emergency room, because she may be having a severe gallbladder attack, and she's worried about picking up Cheerios.

Before I go any further, there is one thing that you must keep in mind when dealing with hospitals, doctors, and nurses. Never, never, never! Accept what you are being told as gospel. If something doesn't seem right, or you feel the doctor has forgotten about a piece of information, then SPEAK UP. Don't be shy about questioning the care provider. Many times they are jumping from patient to patient, and they do forget items from time to time—or sometimes a piece of information isn't conveyed. So don't be afraid of speaking up. They may not like admitting that they forgot something, but they certainly don't want to make a mistake and create an even bigger problem.

Annette was in the emergency room for about three hours, and the physician had done what he could. He ran a few tests that didn't reveal anything significant and was getting ready to release Annette, because the pain was subsiding.

Her pain was subsiding—well, there's a revelation! Do you think it had anything to do with the fact that all the while she was there they were pumping her full of IV painkillers? Annette could have been run over by a tank, and she would have felt no pain. Before the ER doc could discharge her, I frantically called Bill on the phone. I explained to him what was going on, hoping he would be able to stop the ER doc from sending her home. After what seemed like an eternity, the ER doctor hung up the phone with Bill, and Annette was admitted to the hospital.

The next day, we began to run a series of tests. The problem we were running into was that some of the symptoms led in one direction, yet others led in the opposite. The severe pain was saying gallbladder, but the X-rays and CAT scan didn't show any stones. They even scoped her stomach to look for ulcers. No luck.

Somewhere along the line, Annette mentioned to one of the doctors about lifting those boxes in the car three weeks earlier and that she thinks she pulled a muscle or bruised a rib, which very well may be the cause of the pain. Well, just like any other time that information gets passed from person to person, significant little details—like she did this lifting three weeks earlier and there wasn't any pain in the interim—seemed to have evaded some of the doctors. All day long, all we heard was, "Well, there's nothing wrong here. You probably just pulled a muscle." Every time this came up, I would call Bill and tell him that they keep writing in their reports that she pulled a muscle. After about the third call, Bill assured me that we would not be sent home until we knew for sure what was causing the pain.

Near the end of the day, Annette went down for a Hyde scope test. This is where you get to lie still for three hours on a hard, narrow surface about fourteen inches wide while what I would call a type of ultrasound machine watches and records the operation of your gallbladder. Well, what do you know—Annette's gallbladder isn't functioning at all! We watched that darn thing for three hours, and it didn't budge. We thought, Well, that's it, that's the problem. Her gallbladder has gone bad. Back to her room we go.

About an hour later, the surgeon shows up. Annette knows him—not personally, but he was the guy who cut into Dad and Grandma. Dr. Malchik, said, "Well we still don't know for sure if the gallbladder is the culprit, but if you want my opinion, we should yank it."

After a long moment of dead silence and all of us looking at each other, Dr. Malchik continues. With a shrug of his shoulders and anticipating the obvious, he says, "Yes, it is true that this isn't cut-and-dry, but one fact remains: your gallbladder is not functioning."

Once again we found ourselves staring at each other, trying to figure out what the best thing is to do, when Dr. Malchik steps up and says, "Look, it may be the source of the pain and it may not, but it isn't working anyway. The only other option you have is going home and seeing if the pain goes away."

Well, we tried the staying-home-and-seeing-if-it-goes-away routine already. I looked at Annette and said, "You've already done that for three days; it didn't work."

Annette gave me the nod and softly said, "OK," as she closed her eyes. Annette was exhausted, and all she wanted was relief from the pain so she could get some sleep.

That night Annette went under the knife and emerged with four little cuts and one less gallbladder. The next day she seemed fine. The original pain was gone, and they were sending her home to recover.

Armed with Tylenol 3 with codeine for the pain, we went home on the seventh of November. Annette's mother spent the night and was going to stay with her while I was at work the next day.

I got up that morning just as I always did, showered, dressed, and was eager to get back to work. I kissed Annette on the lips and brushed back her hair. She opened her eyes; but this morning she didn't smile. As I caressed her cheek with my hand, I softly asked her how she was feeling.

In a quiet voice she said, "I have a little pain, and I'm itchy all over."

We thought the pain was a normal residual from the operation and kind of blew off the itchiness, thinking it would just pass. In the past, whenever Annette spent the night someplace where it was dry, her skin would itch, so we thought it was from being in the hospital for two days. Hospitals are very dry places.

I kissed her again and told her I would check on her later in the day. It didn't matter where she was or what she wore, Annette was always beautiful to me, especially when she slept. She has this radiance that surrounds her. I loved my work, but I hated leaving every morning even more.

It was about eleven o'clock (there's that time again) when the call came in. Annette was having a reaction to the medicine and was on her way back to the hospital. We should have recognized the symptoms. The itchiness! Annette was having a reaction to the codeine. I say we should have recognized it, because thirteen years ago when Nick was born, Annette had a C-Section, and they gave her Tylenol 3 with codeine, and she had the same reaction. It didn't even dawn on us until we were back at the hospital that night.

This was my first day back after being gone for three days. I sat for a minute debating whether I should go to the hospital or wait and go a little later after getting some work done. But I knew I had to go. I don't know why I felt I had to justify leaving; I'm in charge. It's not like I had to ask permission to leave. Besides, I'm paid a salary that is based on a forty-hour week, and I easily put in sixty to sixty-five hours a week. I don't have to justify anything.

On my way out the door I was running off a list of instructions to whoever was listening when someone shouted out, "JUST GO!" I don't know if they were telling me to go out of concern for Annette or if they were just tired of listening to me and wanted me to get the heck out of their hair. In either case, I am glad they are there to back me up. At their request, I left and headed for the hospital.

I went right into the emergency room to find her, and this time she was there. Of course, her mother was with her, so that eliminated the need to stop and visit on the way.

When I found Annette, they were getting ready to admit her and take her to a room. When you have a reaction to your medication, hospitals don't let you go until they know you are stable. This means the pain has to be under control, and you are eating and functioning (with all things considered) normally.

While Annette was in the hospital, Bill called. He was concerned that Annette may get pneumonia again. It had been almost a week now that she had been flat on her back, and he was worried that she may develop pneumonia. She had a serious case last year at this time, and he wanted to make sure it hadn't returned, so he ordered a chest X-ray. Annette had an X-ray taken two days earlier; I remember standing in the hall outside of the X-ray room waiting for her. It was the morning of her operation; I remember them doing it. But something got screwed up in radiology— they didn't have any film, and there wasn't any record of it. Someone told me later on that one of the radiation technicians was either fired or quit the day Annette had her first X-ray— who knows, maybe this had something to do with the missing film.

Annette didn't go for the X-ray until late on the ninth of November. This was day two of the second stay. The next morning, Bill stopped in with the results of the chest X-ray.

He looked at Annette and said, "They found spots on your lung. They're thinking they are blood clots."

"Blood clots?" I asked.

Bill nodded his head and kind of raised his eyebrows and said, "Well there are three spots, and they suspect they are clots. So until we know what's going on, you aren't leaving. Settle in and make yourself as comfortable as you can. This is going to take a few days. Once we confirm that these are clots, we're going to start you on Heparin and Coumadin and, in the meantime, run more tests to see where the clots are coming from."

Just as before, things didn't add up. The doctors could not determine from the test results where the clots were coming from. The good news was that they were in her lungs. Not that having blood clots in your lungs is a good thing. It's the fact that once the clots make it into the lungs they cannot get out. Clots are formed from two different areas in the body. If they come from your legs they can travel through the arteries into the brain and cause a stroke. Prolonged sitting or being immobile, such as being hospitalized or something as common as being on a plane for four hours, can create clots. This is why it is so important to get up and stretch your legs. Go for a short walk. This eliminated the possibility of one going to the brain and causing a stroke. The other area (which I'm not exactly sure where it is in the body) creates clots and sends them along the left side of your body's arterial system, and they end up in your lungs. So at least it was a slight relief that the clots weren't coming from her legs, which eliminated the chance of a stroke.

It wasn't until the twelfth that that her blood was therapeutic (thinned) and her pain was well enough under control that we could go home, again.

This time I was able to work for two days before getting the call at work.

"Rocco, it's Annette. She's on one." Lisa calls out from the outer office.

"Hi, honey," I answered.

"The pain is real bad, Roc. What should I do?" Annette asked.

I could hear the pain in her voice and feel the tears as they were rolling down her face. I was only leaving her alone for an hour before Kim arrived to be with her while I was at work. I couldn't believe it struck so suddenly and with such force.

"I'll call Kim now and have her come and take you to the hospital."

Kim, her husband Mike, and their three girls moved here from England two years earlier. Kim and Annette became very good friends instantly.

I rang Kim immediately. "Hello, Kim? It's Rocco."

"Oh, yes, Rocco. How are you?" That's how Kim answers the phone.

"Kim," I said. "Annette is in severe pain. Can you please take her to the hospital, and I will meet you there."

"Yes, yes, absolutely. I'll fetch my keys and have her there in a jif." Kim replied.

"Oh, and, Kim. Please don't let her convince you to stop at her mother's."

My next call was to Annette's mom. I knew she would want to be there.

I thought maybe another clot was on the move, and I wanted to see if we could track it. No such luck. After four hours in the emergency room and two tests, the results didn't reveal a thing. The doctor came in and said the tests were all negative.

"It's been a few days since Annette was in the hospital, so naturally her blood counts, sugar counts, and other vital statistics were not up to snuff. I'm looking at the entire picture here," the doctor says. "Because your vitals are a little off, and we need to get this pain under control, we're going to be admitting you (there's a surprise) until we can get you stable."

By now we're getting to know the hospital staff pretty well. You know you've stayed too long when everyone, from the doctors to the transport personnel, knows you by name. As usual, it was Friday, and unless you have an emergency, you wait until Monday before you can get started. So there we sat, trying to put all the pieces together, trying to find some logical explanation. How can you go from being perfectly healthy to this? Why can't the doctors figure out what's wrong? Needless to say, it was a very long weekend.

On Sunday we discussed whether I should stay with her Monday while they ran their tests, like I had done in the past, or if I should go to work and come by later in the day. Thinking that the test results wouldn't be in until late Monday or even Tuesday morning, Annette and I agreed that I should go to work.

It's a tough decision. Do I stay and comfort my wife or go back to work and keep an income coming in and stay active on the insurance plan? At first you want to stay; that's the natural decision. Unfortunately, most people don't have a choice—going to work is a must, and they don't have an option. The reality is (and I'm not picking on large corporations) that the gas company couldn't care less about you and your troubles. You used the gas, and they expect to be paid for it. And I have no grudges there. It's just a fact of life. I'm sure they would work with you if you have been a good customer and paid your bills on time. It's not just the gas company. There's the mortgage, food, lights, water . . . all of the necessities. The bills need to be paid.

Annette and I are extremely fortunate to have a choice. Annette's ability to save money and my determination to provide a steady income has enabled us to build a financial base that will allow me to stay with her during this journey.

We're told that we are lucky to be able to do this. The fact is, luck has nothing to do with it. I don't like to use the word lucky. I think people who rely on luck will never reach that point in their lives where they want to be. About fifteen years ago while I was in the shower, this saying popped in my head, and all of a sudden, things became very clear as to how I was going to achieve my goal of security, both financially and spiritually. It goes like this:

Do not wish me luck, for I do not need luck to survive.
I will succeed on my character and merit.

And that's truly how I feel. The person who counts on luck may survive, but they will never succeed in accomplishing their goals. The other thing that I don't like is the assumption that I have a boss. You will never hear me say "This is my boss" or "I'll have to ask my boss." To me, the only people who have a boss are those who cannot think for themselves and who have to have someone directing them the entire way. I work at a company and there are two owners. There may even be a supervisor or manager, but never a boss. I don't mean to offend anyone; the term boss has become a common reference to the person in charge. If you think about it, though, you really don't need someone to guide you through your work day. You may need to know the direction that they want any project to go or what the goal is, but you don't need someone standing over your shoulder to reach the goal. And that's what a boss does. They oversee your day, minute by minute.

Anyway, getting back to what I was saying. It is a tough decision most have to make. We are fortunate, though. I have worked for a place called All Temp Heating and Cooling for thirteen years, and they have been very supportive, allowing me the freedom to decide whether to come to work or stay with Annette; whichever way I decided they assured me we would be covered. Would they do this for everyone? Maybe. Maybe not. It was my goal, though, to establish a relationship with my employer that regardless of the circumstances I would be able to count on them for their support. They have, and I'm very appreciative. I knew the day would come—I just didn't think it would have come so early in our lives.

Monday morning, eleven forty-five, the phone rings. (I'm really beginning to hate this time of the day.) It's Bill.
"Roc," he says. "You need to come in. I have Annette's test results."
"What's up?" I asked?
"I'd rather talk to you in person," he says.

15

"Just tell me!" I exclaimed.

"We really should do this in person," he said.

"Look, Bill. I don't need to be worried about this all the way to the hospital. Please, I'm asking you nicely. Just tell me."

He starts off with, "Are you sitting down?"

I thought, "Oh, man! This is not going to be good."

"Roc," Bill said, "Annette has cancer."

"What do you mean?" I ask. The correct answer to that question is, What the heck do you think I mean?! but Bill, being the person he is, went on to explain that they had done a CAT scan earlier that morning, and it showed that the spots on her lungs were growths of some sort, and they have multiplied. She now has ten spots; he called them emboli.

"Are you sure it's cancer?" I asked.

"Roc, this could be one of two things," Bill said. "The first thing is, it could be an infection."

"Well, that's not so bad, is it? How do you know it's not an infection?" I replied.

"No, an infection isn't so bad," bill said. "The problem is, her white-blood-cell count isn't up, and it should be skyrocketing with an infection this large."

I fell silent. Suddenly, I was in a world of confusion. My mind was racing; my hands began to tremble.

Bill hesitated a moment and then said in a solemn voice, "It's cancer, Roc. Something is showering her lungs with cancer cells. I'm sorry to have to tell you this, but that's exactly what I think is happening."

"Roc, do you need a ride to the hospital?" Bill asked.

"No . . . No, I'll be OK to drive," I replied.

I was devastated. Every other time when I received the call at work I was out of there in minutes—this time, I just sat there. Rick, one of the owners, was watching while I was on the phone and saw me slide down in my chair. After a minute he came over, took the phone from my hand, hung it up, and asked, "What's wrong?"

I didn't say anything at first; the words wouldn't come out.

Then he asked again. "What's wrong? Is it Annette? Is everything OK?"

After a moment, with a shaky voice, I said, "Umm, they think Annette has cancer."

He sat down without saying a word. "How do they know?" he asked.

"I don't know, but I'm sure they wouldn't be telling me this on a guess."

I have a pretty close relationship with the owners Rick and Tom, and they know Annette well. I knew I wouldn't be back soon. With tears running down my face, I started organizing what work had to be done and what didn't, when Rick came up and said excitedly, "JUST STOP!" As he grabbed my arm at the wrist, looking me square in the eye, he says, "Leave it. Go. We will handle it. Go to the hospital. Don't worry about this." Then he asked, "Do you need a ride?"

"No, I'll be fine. I'll call you when I know more." and I left.

On the way to the hospital, I called Kim.

"Hello, Kim? It's Rocco." With tears running down my face I tell her. "Kim, Annette has cancer."

Kim begins to cry, "Oh, dear Rocco . . . oh no, this can't be," she says.

I could feel her pain. I had to lower the phone from my ear in order to gain my composure before I caused a car accident.

After Kim stopped crying, I said to her, "I need someone to be home for the boys. I don't expect to be coming home from the hospital anytime soon."

"You concern yourself with Annette, and I will care for the boys," Kim said.

I don't remember driving to the hospital . . . I just remember the look on Annette's face when I walked in her room. She was crying, with a look of complete horror in her eyes. There were three people in her room when I arrived, and they all left so we could be alone.

The first thing she said was, "I love you, and I want you to know that you have made me very happy, and I wouldn't have changed a thing."

We hugged and cried and hugged some more. It was very strange. All of a sudden, a thousand things seemed so important . . . so many things to do in a very short period of time. Yet, all we wanted to do was hold each other. Soon, a lady came in with a brochure about cancer and the phone

17

number to the local support group, and that's when it hit us: We need to slow down right now! We didn't even know what kind of cancer Annette has, and this lady is coming in with information. I'll bet I wasn't at the hospital for twenty minutes. It was time to regroup and slow down. If we were going to conquer the beast, we needed to get all the information. If nothing else, it made us feel as if we had taken some type of control over the situation.

Then the big news came. The oncologist at the hospital, an aged gray-haired gentleman (that's what you want when dealing with something like this. You want the guy that has been around awhile. You want what is referred to as a "gray hair"; we would learn later that this isn't always the case), came in, did his exam, talked to Annette and me for a while, and excused himself, stating he would return shortly.

When the doctor came back he stood over Annette and said, "I'm not sure what is wrong with you, but I do know it isn't cancer."

It isn't cancer? I thought to myself. Holy cow, what is going on here? I was elated to hear that Annette didn't have cancer, but I just couldn't believe that Bill would just throw that word around if he wasn't certain.

So I asked the oncologist, "What do you mean it isn't cancer?"

"Cancer doesn't spread this quickly, you haven't been sick enough to indicate that there is anything going on, and, thirdly, the numbers don't add up to cancer."

What numbers? I thought. We had no idea what he was talking about, but we didn't care. We were ecstatic. We couldn't believe our ears. All of a sudden, it didn't matter anymore what Annette had. All we knew was that we would deal with it. We had our life back. All of our dreams were still alive. I honestly don't ever remember being as happy as I was right then and there at any other point in my life. All those happy days—like your wedding day or when your children are born—those days that you would call off when someone would ask, "What was the happiest day of your life?" . . . they couldn't compare to what we felt at that moment.

We kissed each other like we never kissed before. We kissed and held each other as though we had been finally reunited after being separated and jailed by an evil dictator for years. I looked in her eyes and I could feel her love warm my soul. All we wanted to do was make love to each other.

Too bad there was someone in the next bed. That didn't keep Annette from asking.

"Do you want to?" she asks with that smile of hers.

And the lady in the next bed didn't stop me from getting a devilish grin on my face or keep my eyes from lighting up. I went to close the curtain around her bed in a very comical matter when she whispered, "Nooo! We can't."

"Yes, we can," I said as I walked back to her bed.

I climbed in and began kissing her. That's when she lost it. Annette started giggling so loud. It was so wonderful to see her happy; for a brief moment our love had blocked out the pain. A few moments later we were brought back to reality when the nurse came in to check on the patient in the next bed. Annette's roommate was an elderly woman, well-kept and sharp. When the nurse left, I got up to get Annette a glass of water. As I passed Annette's roommate, I greeted her good morning.

Her response was, "Honey, you two should have!"

All three of us laughed. Of all the roommates Annette ended up having, she was the best.

With the oncologist dismissing the possibility of cancer, all of the focus was put on the infection; even though the test results didn't add up to infection. The oncologist was so certain that it wasn't cancer that everyone started trying to make the results fit the diagnosis, instead of letting the diagnosis be the sum of the test results. Annette spent the next twelve days in the hospital. She was given IV antibiotics to try and get the "infection" under control, all the while undergoing every possible test you could imagine. She had X-rays, upper and lower *GI's*, CAT scans and echocardiograms— not to mention she donated about two gallons of blood. Finally a biopsy of the large mass along her abdominal wall, the result of which determined that the mass was a large blood clot. Even after all of this, they still couldn't identify the infection that, according to the doctors, was rapidly growing in her lungs and heart.

This, to say the least, was very disturbing to me. Annette had been on antibiotics for close to twelve days, and I would have at least expected the infection to slow down, if not altogether stop growing. I certainly didn't like the fact that it was still spreading.

I asked Bill, "What's the deal here? Why is this thing still growing?"

Bill's first response was, "These things take time. You have to give the medicine time to work."

I looked at him a little cross-eyed, and I said, "I thought this was supposed to be the best stuff out there." Again I asked, "Why aren't the drugs working?"

He hesitated for a moment and then said, "I still think it's cancer."

This is where I feel we screwed up—we being Bill and I. This is where we should have gone for a second opinion, with the focus being on cancer. But we decided to keep her on IV medication, get her stable, and bring her home.

After the PICC line was installed. (A PICC line is a tube that is inserted into your vein. It will range in length, and Annette's went from her elbow up through her arm and stopped just above her heart. It is used as an IV port to administer medication.) Annette's infectious-disease doctor set her up with Unasyn and Gentamicin. These two drugs are used to treat about 90 percent of all the infections out there successfully. So even though they couldn't identify the infection, this regimen should treat whatever it was that was growing inside her.

Our release from the hospital was delayed a day because Annette's PICC line plugged up. This left us going home the day before Thanksgiving. We had a quiet Thanksgiving at home. Annette was feeling good, as she should, being home for the first time in twelve days.

My angel's comfort was short-lived. Friday morning came with serious nausea. This continued all day Saturday and into Sunday. Bill called to say he was on his way over, and I explained that Annette was still sick.

Bill asked, "Are you giving her the medicine?"

"Yeah," I responded. I thought to myself, What kind of question is that?

Then he quickly followed with, "When are you giving it?"

"As soon as she asks for it. Why?" I asked.

"That's too late," Bill said.

"What do you mean?" I asked.

Bill then explained, "By the time Annette asks for pain relief, the pain has triggered the nausea." Once the nausea kicked in, she couldn't take the pills for pain or the nausea.

It was at this moment that the reality of this thing was kicking in. Up to this point I didn't really grasp the severity of her illness. What I mean to say is, a person reacts in a way that is directly related to their experiences. My experiences with illness like many of us didn't go beyond the common cold or flu. The type of illnesses that you treat after the symptoms arrive. I realized then that I had to change my entire thought process. I had to anticipate where her illness may be headed, I had to start looking for clues, that would help me, help her. I had to be able to recognize if Annette was starting to get dehydrated or disoriented. I had to be able to distinguish the level of pain she was encountering just by her actions or lack of. At one point Annette would sleep more as the pain worsened, her body was doing what it had to in order to keep from going into shock. I became very aware of her every movement. How long she slept, was her speech slurred? Was she attentive when she was awake? Was she eating enough or drinking enough? Not even knowing yet that Annette had cancer.

After understanding the process, we put together a dose schedule that administered the medication in anticipation of the pain, which, in turn, controlled the nausea. Another battle won. At least that's what I thought. Little did I know that this was equivalent to the day before Pearl Harbor.

Monday, December 2, one month since the pain began. By this time, everyone—and I mean everyone—was becoming very concerned. Why is Annette still sick? What do the doctors say? The questions kept coming, and I really didn't have an answer. Then the advice came. Everyone has advice. Some were subtle; others were more direct. The one common piece of advice that we were given was, "You need to go to a different hospital and get a second opinion." Well, it would have been, by now, a third or even a fourth opinion. In our area, there are several hospitals in the immediate area. Many of the doctors are on staff at more than one hospital, so to transfer to a different facility would not necessarily get you a different doctor. On top of this, many of the doctors today work in what they call groups or teams. There are as many as ten doctors in each group.

The doctors spend a great deal of time discussing with their colleagues the more rare cases, and Annette definitely fit that bill. Even though we were at a relatively small hospital, Annette's doctors were members of these groups and on staff at the more prestigious hospitals in the area. So to move on our own just didn't make sense. We were at a small hospital, so she received more attentive care, yet because of the rarity of her case, she attracted the better doctors from the larger hospitals.

I awoke Monday morning before Annette. In anticipation of going to work, I jumped in the shower, shaved, and got dressed. Annette was still quite groggy, so I brought a folding chair upstairs to the bedroom so I could sit next to her. One of the things I always treasured was watching Annette sleep. She sleeps so peacefully and serenely. As I looked at her, the tragedy of all her suffering began to bore deep into my soul. So fragile, so tiny. This "infection" had invaded her body and taken all of the strength and joy that Annette brought to each new day and just discarded it like an old newspaper. As the tears began to roll down my face, I couldn't help but admire the determination my beautiful wife was displaying as she battled this horrid invader. I just wanted to hold her. I wanted to protect her from the villain that was stealing her life away. Yet, there wasn't anything else I could do. We were placing our hopes in God that he would send the best doctors armed with the knowledge and training to face down and conquer this evil aggressor. As I was wiping the tears from my face; Annette woke and placed her hand on my knee.

"Honey," she said.

"Good morning," I replied as I wiped my face.

"I have to go to the bathroom," she whispered softly.

"OK," I said. "We have to take it slow, though. Don't forget you're all wired up here."

When I finished getting her ready for the day, my first question was, "How is the nausea?"

"It's gone," she said, "but I have a lot of pain in my back below my left shoulder."

I didn't say anything but I was very concerned. This was the first time she mentioned any pain in her back. Annette was in pain from the very beginning but never complained about it. I knew if she was telling me about it, it had to be bad. My heart sank. It seemed that every day things just got worse.

Annette could still walk at this time. She was slumped over and needed help, but she was still strong enough to make it down the steps to the loveseat where she spent most of the day sleeping.

We were expecting John that morning. He is a longtime friend of ours, and he was coming in from Chicago to stay for the week and take care of Annette and the boys while I was at work. John is a pharmaceutical rep. I was glad he was coming, not only because he could handle the boys, but with his background, it made it easier to understand some of the thought processes that the doctors were going through. So I made Annette comfortable and told her, "Lets wait and see what the nurse says." The nurse was also coming that morning to do her weekly exam.

The initial plan was to get Annette up, have the nurse come and do her thing, and then cut out and go to work, leaving Annette with John. Well, as it turned out, the nurse was very concerned about the pain; she thought there was a concern that Annette was bleeding internally and that we should call the doctor to see if they wanted Annette to come in for an X-ray. I called Bill to let him know what was going on. I told him the nurse said to call Annette's surgeon.

Bill said, "No, you probably want to call Annette's infectious-disease doctor."

I called the surgeon any way. The nurse at the surgeons office said, that most likely it's not something that was caused by the surgery, and it would be a waste of time to bring her to them, not to mention, the strain it would put Annette, driving all over town unnecessarily. They felt I should call the lung doctor. So I called the lung doctor. They said the same thing the surgeon said and suggested I call the infectious-disease doctor. I called and they said to bring her in to the hospital for an X-ray. When I saw Bill at the hospital, I told him about the fiasco I created earlier on the phone.

He put his head down, looked over his glasses, and said, "Roc."

I knew what he meant immediately, but sometimes you just have to go your own route. Bill's a smart guy, and he's very good at diagnosing problems. I don't know why I just didn't listen to him and call the infectious-disease doc first off. I guess sometimes I do or say something just to let that person know that I'm looking over their shoulder and questioning what they are saying or doing. It's something I learned to do so the person you're dealing with stays focused.

John arrived about nine o'clock that morning. Annette wasn't in any condition for traveling; she was tired and sore from the PICC line, and she was doped up pretty good from the medication. But I dressed her and made our way back to the hospital. By now it was almost noon. It was a miracle, the timing of John coming that morning. Little did we know that John just went from lending a hand to becoming a surrogate parent for the next week. We didn't wait very long before she went for the X-ray, and it wasn't very long before Bill came out and said, "We are admitting Annette back into the hospital; the infection is spreading."

I was devastated. Here we had been treating Annette with the best IV antibiotic drugs since the twelfth of November, and this thing was still growing.

I couldn't stay with her that night. There was no way I could leave the boys with someone else again. For the last month, every time Annette went in to the hospital or doctor's office, she didn't come home for at least a week. Even though John was a close friend and the boys really enjoy it when John and Tammy and their four girls come for a visit, I couldn't disappear on them again. I can't imagine what is going through their minds right now. They have been very strong up to this point, seeing their mom stricken down with illness and living out of suitcases week after week as they are shuffled from house to house every time Annette is admitted back into the hospital. These same boys that would drive you nuts with their constant jousting had put all that aside and allowed me to concentrate on helping their mom get better. I will probably say this more than once, but it is worth saying a hundred times: KIDS GET IT! Don't underestimate kids; they are more in-tuned to what is really important than most adults.

I left the hospital about nine that night. I called Tom at home to let him know I wouldn't be into work the next day, and I didn't know how long I would be gone. I couldn't tell you how many days I had missed prior to this, but Tom said to just do what I had to do and they would be OK. He also added, "You need to get her somewhere else." He even offered to come that night and break her out of there. That was a little extreme, but he was right. I know I talked about the hospitals and how the doctors were on staff at multiple facilities, but this wasn't working.

I didn't sleep that night. The next day I returned to the hospital as soon as I got the boys off to school. I know I haven't mentioned this up to this point, but so you can start to try to understand the circumstances that fueled our frustration and fears. You have to realize that Annette turned forty in April, I'm forty-two, and our boys are nine, eleven, and thirteen. She's too young for this. She has so much more life ahead of her. When I look at Annette and feel the helplessness; I can only wonder; how it is for the parents of a small child that has cancer. To watch your child suffer the pain and not be able to do anything about it; the thought is so incomprehensible, I don't know what words to use to explain to you what I'm feeling right now.

I returned to the hospital with a vengeance that morning. As soon as I made it to the room I was on the phone with the shop. I'm in the heating and cooling industry. I started out doing service, went into sales, and worked my way to general manager. Along the way, I built a fairly large base of customers, some of whom I would consider friends. Of those people, a few were doctors. I called the shop to get phone numbers, and I started calling around to see if any of them could help us. The response was overwhelming. I had wives calling their husbands, mothers calling their sons and daughters—all of whom were doctors—and, in turn, they were calling their colleagues. All these people dropped what they were doing right then and there to help us. Within minutes I was receiving responses and suggestions back from all over the state. Some were helpful, and some called to say it was out of their field but wanted to leave their name and number in case I needed anything down the road. To this day I am overwhelmed by the generosity of strangers. I knew these people's parents or friends, but I didn't know them—yet they were reaching out to help if they could. I always believed there is much more good in this world than bad, and that morning brought it home.

25

Shortly after the phone stopped ringing, Annette's doctor came into the room. This was unusual; typically she didn't make her rounds until later in the afternoon, but today she showed up early. Not a good sign. She went on to explain that she was going to order a biopsy of one of the growths in Annette's lung. YES! I jumped up and raised my fist in the air victoriously. Annette's infectious-disease doctor had been talking about doing this for a while, but the lung docs had been resisting it. Because of the risk whenever you puncture the lung, the consensus was to leave doing a biopsy of the growth in the lung as a last resort.

During the last stint in the hospital they did an echocardiogram of the right side of Annette's heart. This showed what they call vegetation on the right bicuspid valve. Because of the location of this vegetation, it could not be successfully treated with antibiotics. In other words, the drugs could not reach the valve and kill off the bacteria. This is what they felt was creating all of the problems.

The doctor then asked, "Where would you like to go to have heart surgery, if it comes to that?"

"What are our choices?" I asked.

Her response was Kensington Hospital or one of the local hospitals that specialized in heart surgery.

I asked, "If it was your daughter, where would you take her?"

"To Kensington Hospital," she replied.

I was a little surprised at that answer, because she was on staff at one of the more prestigious hospitals that specialized in cardiac care.

She then explained that the best doctors at her hospital were trained by the doctors at Kensington Hospital.

At this point, I thought that making the move would be based on the results of the biopsy. Later that day when Annette went in for the biopsy, the doctor came right out of the room and asked if we had decided what hospital we wanted to go to.

I jumped right on it and said, "Kensington Hospital!"

I certainly wasn't thrilled that Annette was going for heart surgery. But, once again, I felt we were moving in a forward direction. For what seemed like an eternity, we weren't progressing in the treatment. We were stagnant, and no one really knew what direction they wanted to go. No one knew because we had the right doctors treating the wrong diagnosis. It all goes back to when the first oncologist said, and I quote, "I'm not sure what you have, but I'm sure it's not cancer." That statement threw Annette into the lap of an exceptionally talented infectious-disease doctor. She was doing all she could with what was available to her, yet here we were still fighting our way through the hedge row. In a way I felt bad for her. Everyone was looking to her for answers—answers to a question that wasn't meant to be. I knew and she knew that something wasn't right. In fact, every time we saw her, part of her visit included a brief conversation where she reiterated that what she was seeing still didn't convince her that Annette had an infection and that maybe there was something else going on. In spite of this, she kept giving Annette all she had. She never gave up on her.

What a great relief, though; the decision to transfer Annette was the doctor's and not mine. One of the hardest things that you have to deal with is having to make a decision about treatment on your own. Things certainly weren't going well up until now, but who's to say that moving Annette was going to make any difference? You hear stories of how people take matters into their own hands, but you only hear of the ones that have happy endings. I can't recall being told or seeing a story on the news when it didn't work out for the better. Like everything else in this world, for every one success there has to be at least two failures. This may be a little pessimistic, especially for someone like myself who always tries to find the positive side of a situation. I just can't believe that an uneducated guess is equal in results to an informed decision. That's right, a guess. I don't care how much you research something; if you're an amateur in that field, all you're doing is guessing; you can't possibly know what you don't know. And if you don't have all of the information then you are just guessing;— an extremely critical guess, I may add. Every time people (meaning your family and friends) hear that the doctors don't have a definite fix on the problem, they all start looking at you to do something about it. I'll get into this a little later on, because this belongs in a section all by itself. Anyway, it was a relief to me that the doctor recommended transferring Annette and that we were finally moving ahead.

Later on, it dawned on me. The biopsy had nothing to do with transferring Annette; it hadn't even made it to the lab before the doctor came out asking if we had decided on a hospital. She already knew before Annette went in that she was a candidate for surgery. What were they looking for? Once again, the doctor briefly led on that this may not be an infection at all, but I guess I chose to ignore that because the alternative was cancer.

Have you ever been transferred from a small local hospital to a large research hospital such as Kensington? Annette's biopsy was on Tuesday. We finally made it to Kensington Hospital on Thursday evening. The first thing that has to happen is your doctor has to request a transfer. Then the doctors at Kensington Hospital review the case. Once a doctor accepts the case (I had no doubt that they would; all along they have been telling us how rare Annette's case was, and if there was one thing Kensington Hospital is looking for, it's a rare case), it then goes to admitting at the hospital. Once they check out your insurance and locate a bed for you, they contact your hospital and arrangements are made to transfer you. This took two days. It felt like two months. In the meantime, Annette spent a great deal of time sleeping, but while she was awake, we would talk and even managed to get in a game of cards.

On Thursday, December 4 at five o'clock, we were on the move. Our spirits were high; we felt it was the beginning of the end. Bill had taken me around the hospital earlier that day to collect all of Annette's records, X-rays, and CAT scans. Bill instructed to hand-carry the records and hold to on to them until I could personally hand them to the doctor, and so I did.

My mother-in-law and I reached the hospital shortly after the ambulance. When we got to my wife's room, she was just getting settled in. They're very efficient at Kensington Hospital. Within minutes, two nurses came in, a lady from the kitchen came by with some food, and the physician's assistant came in to interview Annette and get her history. He also made sure she was comfortable and that we understood what the next steps would be. I could see peace in Annette's eyes; I held her hand and kissed her forehead. I whispered "I love you" in her ear, and she gently squeezed my hand as she drifted off to sleep.

Mom and I left for the hotel that night feeling very good. Annette was in the best hands, the best minds, and one of the best facilities in the nation, if not the world. I was pumped; I was going to do anything I had to in order to keep the ball rolling.

The following morning we were at the hospital by six. I didn't want to miss the doctor. We waited until nine, and the doctor still hadn't come. Annette insisted that we go get some breakfast. I didn't want to go, but my mother-in-law needed to eat, and the nurse couldn't tell us if the doctor was coming or not, so we went to the cafeteria. Well, guess what? Yeah, you guessed it. The doctor came while we were gone. I didn't miss him by much, so I went looking. I spotted him down the hall, so I stopped him and introduced myself. He was described to me as a kind man with a great bedside manner. I have to say that was very true. He took the time to explain that he is going to order another CAT scan, chest X-ray, and an echocardiogram. He also told me he needed the videotape of Annette's last echocardiogram.

I've been there for all of Annette's other tests, so I knew I didn't have to be there for this round—I would just be standing around. Besides, her mother was there, so I wasn't concerned. Why should I be? This was the beginning of the end. It was all downhill from here. So I volunteered to go and get the videotape from the first hospital. Not only did it speed up the process by a day or two, not having to wait for the tape to arrive by courier, but it gave me an excuse to get out of the hospital, which by now was becoming very old.

The hospital wouldn't have the tape until later that afternoon, so I hung around Kensington Hospital for a while. Just before I left, the charge nurse came in and said they were moving Annette to a private room. She said this would make it easier if I had decided to stay the night. I didn't pay much attention to this kind gesture; I just thought the nurse was trying to be nice. Annette's new room had a nice view looking over the hospital grounds. Right outside her window was a court yard filled with flower beds that I'm sure created a beautifully serene environment during the summer months. Circling the flowerbeds was a brick-pavers pathway with benches placed along its edge. Shortly after we settled Annette into her new room, I brushed back her hair and kissed her forehead, gently squeezing her hand. I whispered in her ear that I loved her and that I would be back before she returned from her tests.

Implosion

I was on the expressway heading back to Kensington Hospital when my cell phone rang. It was Bill.

"Roc, where are you at?" he asked.

"I'm driving back to Annette," I replied.

"Yes, I know, but where exactly are you now?"

"I'm on the expressway. I-75 and 12 Mile Rd."

Then Bill says, "Pull over."

"Why?" I asked.

"Just pull over!" Bill exclaimed.

"OK, OK, I've stopped. Now tell me what's up."

"I have the results from the biopsy," Bill said. After a slight hesitation, he choked out the phrase, "Roc, it's cancer, just as I suspected. Annette has cancer."

I put the van in park and just sat there. Our fears have come to be. For the second time in a five-week span, our world imploded. It was strange, though. I didn't react this time the way I did the first time. I think deep down inside I knew this was more than just an infection. Bill offered to come and get me and drive me back. But I was convinced that I was alright to drive, and after the best sales pitch in my life, I convinced Bill that I was OK to drive.

When I returned to Annette's room, not ready to face her with the news, I glanced in before entering. Her mom was there alone, anxiously pacing the room.

"Mom" I called out as I walked in.

She turned and said that Bill called looking for me. I told her that I know; in fact, I had just talked to him. After a brief pause I placed my hand on her shoulder and, looking her in the eye, I told her she needed to sit down. It's strange, under circumstances like this, when someone tells you to sit down you know it can't be good, so you continue to stand like this feeble act of defiance is going to change the inevitable. Once she was seated, I broke the news to her. She totally lost it. Grace broke out into a panic. She began crying as the pain poured out from deep inside her. Her grief had risen so quickly she began flailing her hands indiscriminately.

She was so out of control I had to restrain her from hitting herself in the head.

With today's media coverage you can witness from afar the anguish of those who have faced the demon of fear. Never before have I witnessed the emotion firsthand. It travels through the room just as a strong wind gusts through an open window. This is when it hit me. My wife—the woman I adored for twenty years and shared a loving marriage of over eighteen years . . . forty years old and the mother of our three boys—has cancer. Our world was crashing in, and she didn't even know it yet. The next ten minutes seemed like an hour. This phenomenon of time standing still would become a torturous piece of this entire puzzle.

We had just enough time to gain our composure before Annette returned to the room. She was sedated pretty well, so she didn't notice how somber the room was. I caught Dr. Miller, Annette's heart surgeon, before he entered the room. Dr. Miller is a very thin man that stands over six feet tall. I looked up and told him that I had received a phone call with the results of the biopsy from Annette's lung, and it revealed that she has cancer. At the time, we were standing right in the doorway of Annette's room, so he swept me into the guest lounge, which just happened to be right next door.

He said that this had confirmed what he had been seeing. Then he went on to explain. The echocardiogram did not show any growth on the heart valve; in fact, it showed the valve to be in very good condition. He suspected that what they saw was a blood clot. There was a large clot in her heart. Part of it was still in her heart below the valve, and there was another clot in the arterial vein going to her lungs. This piece was more than likely part of the clot in her heart that was sitting on the valve, and now it had broken off and was heading for her lungs. I had a million questions that he couldn't answer. Not that he isn't a good doctor; in fact, it was just the opposite. He is a prominent cardiac surgeon and came highly recommended by his peers; the other patients that we met on the floor praised his skills and bedside manner. It's just that Annette moved from a cardiac patient to an oncology patient. Dr. Miller did convince me that he should be the one to break the news to Annette, and I'm glad he did.

His approach left her feeling strong and determined, where I'm sure mine would have left her with a feeling of despair.

Dr. Miller sat next to Annette's bed, calling her name as he gently rubbed her shoulder to bring her out of the sedation. In a kind and soothing voice he explained to her that her valve was in good condition; in fact, her heart as a whole was very healthy. The doctor then proceeded to tell her that the biopsy showed that she had cancer. Not being an oncologist and not having all of the information, he couldn't give her any more information about it. He did encourage her, though, by ensuring her that other than the cancer, she was in very good condition. This gave Annette the spirit to prepare for a battle. A battle against uncertainty and fear.

As soon as Dr. Miller left, I started making phone calls. The first person I called was Annette's brother Sam. When I first met Sam, he was very young; I believe he was still in middle school . . . sixth or seventh grade. In fact, if it wasn't for Sam, Annette and I probably wouldn't be married. Sit back now, and I'll tell you how Annette and I met.

Twenty years ago I was asked to stand up in my cousin's wedding. Not only was this unusual because this particular cousin is eight years my senior, but we didn't really have any contact other than family get-togethers on the holidays. As it happened, my cousin's bride-to-be was from a very large family, and the age range of those standing up in the wedding varied greatly. I stood up with Susan who, in turn, was a friend of Annette's. They were from Rochester Hills, which is much different than the small country town that I was from.

As the wedding progressed with parties and rehearsals, I came to know Susan a little better. Susan belonged to a group at her church called the Eleventh Commandment Group. It was a group designed to bring together young people between the ages of eighteen and twenty-five. I forget now how often they met, but for the most part, it was more of a social club than a religious group. Many of the meetings were held at local establishments, such as restaurants and bars. We would go dancing, play volleyball, or just sit around and talk. One time a few of us got together to go horseback riding. (That's a story in itself.) All in all, it was a good time. Anyway,

Susan invited me to come to one of the meetings. I later figured out that she invited me as a courtesy, because she also invited my cousin Mitch, who was also standing up in the wedding. Mitch was definitely more in the groove than I was. Smart, fashionable, and, without a doubt, more of a ladies' man than I was.

Under normal circumstances I would have just passed on the invitation and stayed in my little comfort zone, but I had just broken up with a girl, my teaching position was on the chopping block as a result of tax cuts coming into play, and I recently joined the Air Force. My entire character had changed, so I accepted the invite and started going to the meetings. People talk about fate; well, this is where it really gets strange.

I attended a couple of meetings when it was announced that one of the members was inviting whoever wanted to go to his parent's cottage on Burt Lake. It took a couple days to decide, but I finally found the nerve to sign up to go. At this time, I still didn't know Annette very well, and I couldn't believe that I was going away for the weekend with a bunch of strangers; the old Rocco never in a million years would have done that. I don't know what attracted me to Annette; maybe it's because she is so approachable. She doesn't prejudge you. It didn't matter to her that I still wore cut-off jeans in the world of hemmed shorts made popular by the Magnum P.I. series.

The first day there, everyone decided to go down to the beach. After sitting on the beach talking for about thirty minutes, everyone headed for the water to cool off. Annette is five-foot-nothing and weighs in at one hundred pounds. As the group headed out into the lake, Annette had to stop because the water was up to her neck. When we finally stopped, I turned around to see Annette standing alone about thirty yards behind us. I don't know why, but I went back to where she was standing, and our life together started at that moment. (It's twenty years later, and I can still see her standing there with this big smile on her face.)

To this day, I'm not sure why I went over to be with her. I felt bad that she got left behind, but I was extremely shy around women, and to go one-on-one with someone I knew briefly was really stepping out there.

We spent the entire weekend together and became the item of the trip. I remember the second night when we went for a walk down to the lake and around the neighborhood. We were gone quite awhile. By the time we returned, everyone else was asleep. I said good night and was heading for my bed when I turned around to see Annette standing in the doorway of her bedroom. As I said before, I was pretty shy around women, so I didn't even attempt a good-night kiss. Yeah, this is day two, and after spending all day together, I was still apprehensive about asking for a kiss. But there stood Annette. I walked back over to her.

"Well," she asked, "don't you want to kiss me?"

She didn't wait for my answer. She just wrapped her arms around my neck and planted one right on my lips. She slowly stepped back holding my hand, winked at me, and walked into her room. I stood there for a second before heading back to my room. All I could think of was, how was I going to get to sleep now? The next day, everyone went canoeing. Naturally, Annette and I teamed up in one canoe. It was great; overnight we went from acquaintances to a couple. We talked and laughed as if we'd known each other for years.

I forget the name of the river we canoed, but we had a blast. The current was pretty fast, but the scenery was beautiful. The shoreline was lined with trees and wildflowers. As the river wound through the trees you could hear the water rushing along its edge. The birds were singing, and you could hear everything that was happening on the river, because the sound traveled so far. We could hear our friends up ahead and behind us planning their attack. We quietly listened to their plan and then decided to play coy, allowing them time to come up behind us. We talked and laughed as though we were oblivious to everything around, and as soon as they were within firing range, we unloaded with our paddles, splashing water and drenching everyone in the canoe. This only took a few seconds, and we were roaring with laughter, never really looking behind us to see which group we slaughtered. Taunting them, the fools, to think they could get us, I turned my head to see that Annette and I had drenched a couple and their two small children. After a brief moment of horror, I whimpered out, "I'm sorry, we thought—" and that's when they started laughing. Their kids started their counterattack, and the battle was back on. When all were wet, I handed Dad a beer as they paddled on past us.

The rest of the weekend we were inseparable.

I even met her parents that weekend. You see, Annette's family had a cottage not to far from there. Well, I invited Annette to ride home with us instead of going back with her family. When Annette's mom and dad came to pick her up, I introduced myself and convinced them to let Annette go back with us. Well, I was partially successful; Annette was allowed to go with another group: a car full of girls that was part of the caravan. You see, Annette's parents still carried many of the old-world Italian beliefs about boys and girls. To send their daughter off in a car full of guys just wouldn't sit well. (Let me point out that she was twenty at the time.) Anyway, she was able to go. I even bought her flowers at a roadside stop. Some romantic, wouldn't you say?

The following Monday, without hesitation, I called to talk. We had such a good time over the weekend I never gave a second thought to calling her. Sam answered the phone and said she wasn't home. I called for the next four days and got the same answer. I didn't believe it. I knew her schedule, and I knew she would be home by a certain time. I couldn't believe I was being dumped. Not only was I on the outs, but she wouldn't even talk to me. There I was, outside my comfort zone—an area that I had built so well to keep me safe from all that I couldn't control—and the first time I venture from the cave, I get whacked! She used me, and I couldn't do anything about it.

I don't know why, but I decided to call her one more time. Amazingly enough, Sam answered the phone again! (This was many years before caller ID. This was back to the days that when the phone rang, you had no idea who was on the other end.) After I pleaded with him to have her come to the phone, he told me to wait and he would get her. I waited and waited and waited. I learned later that Sam had to physically take her to the phone and tell her, "Look, at least talk to the guy, so he'll quit calling,"

Once I had Annette on the phone, we talked for at least an hour. We were back to where we left off a week ago. After an hour, it didn't take much to get her to go out on another date; actually, this would have been our first official date. We went to dinner at a Chinese restaurant and, as dinner wound down, as is customary in Chinese restaurants, our waitress brought us our fortune cookies. Annette's read: "The path you follow for true love is shorter than you think." Her mouth fell open, and then she began to blush. Without a sound she passed it to me and held my hand as I read it aloud. When I finished reading it, I looked at Annette, and she couldn't stop smiling. Then I opened my cookie, and it read: "He who walks in the dark stubs his toes." I guess that's better than lucky numbers.

Well, the bill came, but Annette had excused herself to use the ladies' room. Before going, she gave me a coupon for $5 off. Wow, this was great. Tiny, pretty, cute, and frugal—I hit the mother load. I paid the bill, and we walked out of the restaurant.

As we headed for the car, Annette asked, "Did they accept the coupon?"

"Oh, shoot!" I said. I had forgotten to give it to them.

Annette shook her head, took the coupon, went back into the restaurant, and got my $5. Mind you, this is our first date.

That night, I asked her what was up. "Why were you so reluctant to talk to me when I called?"

It turned out that she had been talking to her friends. If you want to screw up a relationship, take advice from friends. I think more times than not they have their own agenda, and it doesn't always have your best interests at heart. A truly good friend, one that will put your needs above their own, are few and far between. And Annette did not have a truly good friend at this time in her life, as she later learned. You see, I was scheduled to leave for the Air Force in three months, and she was advised that a relationship like this would only bring heartbreak to her, and she wasn't going to expose herself to it. It seems that even though these women didn't even know me, it was clear to them that I would cheat on Annette. In their eyes, it was obvious that anyone in the position I was in, being so far away, would take advantage of the distance and be dating other women.

Over the years, I have come to the conclusion that the most suspicious people are the very ones that contemplate doing such deeds. I ask you, who is more suspicious of being cheated and who is more concerned about being ripped off: the thief or the honest person? The thief, of course; they're the person that has figured all of the angles. The honest guy will take a person for their word, not jump to a conclusion of distrust. The person that doesn't trust anyone else is the very person you need to keep a close eye on. Going out with other women never even crossed my mind. So, you see, if it wasn't for Sam, it is very possible that we may not even be together now.

As I said before, Sam was the first person I called. He's single without a family at home to be with. This meant he was the most flexible, and I needed someone to go back to the hotel with Mom. I wasn't leaving Annette's room, and there wasn't enough room for three people to spend the night. Besides, I needed to be alone with her. It dawned on me then that the nurses knew that this was going to turn into more than just another operation, which is why they moved us to a private room.

I don't remember what time all this started that day; I do know it was sometime in the evening. I was falling apart by the second. I called my mother so she would know who, in turn, spread the word through my family. My next call was to friends of ours whose son was diagnosed a couple years earlier with cancer. Just out of dumb luck, Nicole, Annette's long-time friend, had brought Dominic, her son, in for a treatment earlier that day and came up to see Annette. She said she would be back the next day to visit. When Nicole was here earlier Annette hadn't gotten the news about the cancer yet. I felt Nicole should know ahead of time. I didn't want her to walk into the room the next day and get hit in the face with this; she needed to be told ahead of time, so she could prepare. The last thing she needed was to be blindsided with more bad news. Nicole and her family had enough to deal with.

Reality was beginning to kick in. I couldn't focus on a single thought, and it was difficult putting two words together. Needing to get out of the room for a while, I decided to go to the lobby and meet Sam. I always had a snap in my walk. When I was walking somewhere, I walked with a purpose. Poor Annette, being only five feet tall, would have to take two steps to my one to keep up. It wasn't until a few years earlier that I became conscious that she was literally running to keep up with me. That night it was all I could do to keep standing. I finally made it to the lobby where I was supposed to meet Sam.

Anyone who has a spouse and kids and is used to having them around knows that empty feeling you get when you have to leave and go out of town for a few days. There's emptiness there, and it just sits on your chest, causing you to want to give yourself a hug. Well, multiply that by a thousand, and you might begin to understand the agony that was building inside. It's funny how the body and mind have a relief system in place to try and prevent a total shutdown. I sat there on that couch waiting for Sam, and even though I tried, I couldn't stop running all of the scenarios through my mind of what I must have done wrong. This couldn't be happening to us. Oblivious to everything around me, I was trapped in this misty world in my mind where nothing was clear. After a while, I couldn't put two thoughts together. I just sat there like a lump. I remember watching people as they walked by. There was this fuzzy aura around them. Kind of like in a dream you can see what you are looking directly at, but everything else is out of focus and distorted. They were talking and laughing, making plans, telling stories about their day and yelling at their kids for running in the lobby. I remember thinking how truly blessed they were.

Let me tell you about Annette's younger brother. Sam was a guy that always seemed to take life as it came. Never a worry, never a plan. Just ride with the wind and deal with whatever comes when it arrives. If we saw Sam two times a year outside of holiday dinners it would have been a lot. Over the next few months I wouldn't be able to get rid of him. He canceled a cruise to the Bahamas and a trip to Disney World that he was planning with his son. He started doing research, questioning the medical staff, and making himself available for every meeting with the doctors. Sam stepped up to the plate, taking care of the boys while I was at the hospital. I don't know what I would have done in the beginning days without him. When the doctors came to talk, I would follow the conversation for a few minutes and then begin to lose focus as more bad news was being relayed to us. Thank God he was there to help fill in the gaps. Even today all I have to do is pick up the phone, and he will be there to help his sister . . . to help all of us.

Sam showed up at the hospital about eleven thirty that night, and he had brought Annette's sister Joann. By now I was spent. I was emotionally drained, and we hadn't even talked to a doctor from the oncology department yet. I didn't know how bad it was. All I knew was every time we had another test done, the situation became worse.

Sam and Joann literally moved in that night. There is a hotel attached to Kensington Hospital, and earlier that day I made reservations for the next seven days. This way, if anyone wanted to stay, they would have a place to sleep, I never anticipated it would become an oasis where friends and family could go and rest or take a shower while someone else stayed with Annette and me. What a great idea: family members could stay at the hotel and walk to and from the room that their loved one was in without ever going outside. There is a nice cafeteria and a fast-food joint located in the corridor between the hospital and the hotel. After spending over a month in a hospital, it was nice having some variety to choose from, even though we weren't eating much.

The next day we were visited by a "gray hair," an elderly gentleman that made initial visits to patients. I still haven't figured out the exact reason for these visits—they are filled with speculation based on absolutely no medical evidence. By the time he left, all hope for recovery was obliviated. According, to the good doctor, there were multiple nodules, or tumors, that had spread into Annette's breast. (This was new from just the day before when her chest X-ray and CAT scan only showed two nodules; now she had at least ten more.) With this information, he informs us that if she didn't receive treatment immediately, it would be too late. He also felt that Annette, more than likely, had a form of lung cancer. That was a guess, and we knew it. He said he was only guessing, and I could understand that. It was Saturday, and there was no way of getting accurate information from a lab at a different hospital. I just wish he didn't tell us about the increasing growth in Annette's breast. It didn't do us any good knowing that information. It wouldn't change the outcome. Besides, it was a physical exam; it wasn't confirmed by any scan. I didn't understand why he would drop in on a Saturday morning and create such disparity.

I don't have to tell you what the mood in the room was like. All we could picture was this horrid disease running rampant inside her body. Have you ever seen a movie where they use a map to show you how a disease or plague was spreading across the country? It's usually a map of the United States, and in seconds it turns from pasture green to a dingy brown as the plague spreads across the nation. This is all we could picture as to what was happening inside Annette's body. There wasn't a dry eye in the room. Not only did we receive the equivalent of the kiss of death, but it was Saturday morning, and you know what that means: you wait until Monday before you see another doctor. It is one beauty of a system we have. On the one hand, you're told your situation is very bleak. The other is you have to wait because it's the weekend, and the doctors have all gone home. Once again we were left in this land of disbelief, where it just doesn't seem to be real. This can't be happening. We all just sat there waiting for someone to come in and wake us up from this nightmare.

These were the longest two days of my life. The entire time was spent full of pain and tears. Just as it did in the hospital over five weeks ago, the news had severed all of our dreams and plans for the future. All I could think about was spending the rest of my life alone without Annette. She wouldn't be there to see the boys graduate or get married. She wouldn't be there to hold our grandchildren. Our plans of travel when we retired were gone. All the fun we shared going away for the weekend would be no more. Who would I hold on Christmas morning as the boys opened their gifts? There was nowhere to hide. Nothing I did could remove the pain. It is a pain that is indescribable. Never in my wildest dreams did I ever imagine that this kind of pain could even exist. To be so elusive to the touch yet burrowed so far down into your soul that it becomes part of your being.

I remember sitting, staring out the window watching the sun come up. I didn't sleep at all that night, and I just couldn't stop watching Annette. She would sleep so soundly from the medication that her breathing was very soft. And she rarely moved; I found myself constantly checking to see if she was still breathing. This continues still today. I wake two or three times a night to see that she is still with us. How can your life change so drastically in a matter of days? I couldn't stop hurting. I just wanted someone to come in and tell me that everything would be alright. That person never came.

That night while I was watching Annette sleep, my thoughts would bring back memories of all the good times we shared. When I would come home from work, I would come up behind her and give her a hug, or let the back of my hand brush her behind as I walked by. Other times she would be exercising, and when I walked into the room, I would be greeted with a wink and a smile, or her aerobic exercise would turn into a dance with her pointing her finger at me, motioning me to come join her in a sexy dance in the middle of the front room. Annette was always full of life. She made our days bright and full of energy. She has such a lively spirit. To see her now brings tears to my heart. So weak, so fragile. It hurts her to even roll over. Even with everyone coming around I still felt as if Annette and I were the only ones in the room.

Soon, the phone calls started, and people started showing up as the word got out about Annette's diagnosis. All who called or came wanted to help . . . a little too much. I didn't have time to think. They kept asking what, where, and when could they be of help. Would I need help at home or maybe taking her to the doctor? Who would be there to care for the boys? What about work . . . Who do I want to be there when I return to work?

Over the next day and a half I fended off the questions with a simple "I don't know. Why don't you guys tell me when you are available?" I would ask. They didn't know much either.

After a while I just stopped responding and crawled into a corner to be alone. Finally, I left and went to the waiting room to get away. Sam came in a few minutes later, followed by Joann. I looked up, and before I could say anything, Sam said, "We're not here to talk. We just came to sit."

After a few minutes I slowly raised my head and said, "You guys keep asking for me to decide as to who needs to be where and when. Can you tell me how to do that? I've never had to deal with this before. I don't know what her treatments will be or how often or even the effect they will have."

All this time the emotion was building inside, and soon the real question comes to the surface. No longer could I contain or ignore the inevitable question. As the emotion begins to flow and the tears start running down my face, I looked directly into Joann's eyes and asked, "How do I decide how much time is enough to be by Annette's side? Do I go back to work? What if she only lives for two weeks or a month? How do I decide when I don't know what will be? How do I decide how much time to spend with her when we don't even know how serious this is? Annette is sick, and I don't care about work! I want to spend every moment I can with her. Can you please try to understand this?" I shouted.

"This isn't about organization and efficiency. This is about hanging on to every moment as long as possible."

By this time I'm bawling. The grief had overwhelmed me. I fell deep into my chair as groans of agony filled the room. The pain was entrenched, and it was tearing me apart. For the first time in my life, I felt terror and paranoia. My body trembled with pain. I looked frantically around the room. What I was looking for I don't know. Then I felt Joann's arms wrap around me, holding me tight, just as you would hold a terrified child that was awakened by a horrible nightmare. Joann didn't let go until the terror had passed. After that they stopped asking. We spent the rest of that Sunday trying to keep Annette comfortable. She was throwing up a lot and had a terrible case of dry skin, which was very itchy.

Let me take a minute and tell you a little bit about Joann. Being the eldest of the siblings, Joann has taken on the role of overseeing everything that is going on. She has become the planner and organizer. More important, she will become Annette's pillar of spiritual support. Annette's faith in God is very strong, and Joann provided a wealth of energy through prayer. I truly believe the reason Annette has been so strong during this entire journey is because of Joann's ability to give her the spiritual support that she so desperately needs—a need that, at the moment, I cannot fulfill. I love her for that.

Monday morning came. We were anxious for the doctor to come in. Around nine, the doctor and his entourage of physicians and students came into the room.

"Hello. I'm Dr. Mathews, and I feel, without a doubt, that you should be treated at a facility closer to your home."

Holy cow! Not a "How are you feeling?" or "Did you sleep well last night?" The doctor simply announced, "You're in the wrong place, and as soon as we can move you safely, you're out of here." Usually when something like this would happen I would jump all over it, giving the doctor a piece of my mind as to how he could take his opinion and,--well I won't go there. Where is the compassion? What happened to bedside manner? But I was drained, and this was another blow. It took us five weeks just to get here, and now we were being kicked out. At least, that's how I felt at the moment.

Then Dr. Mathews continued. "With that being said, you need to understand that the type of cancer that you have is very difficult to treat." Pulling up a chair, he sat down next to Annette and held her hand. "You have what is known as Carcinoma of unknown primary. This is where a person doesn't have a primary tumor that the cancer cells are coming from. Originally, we thought that this meant that they couldn't find the primary tumor, and it was just a matter of time before we had a handle on the source. We learned later that this is a specific kind of cancer. There is a form of cancer where a tumor sprouts up, spreads its seeds, and dies off. The best comparison that I can think of is it acts like a dandelion. It shoots up quickly, blooms, goes to seed, and dies off, leaving behind hundreds of seeds just waiting to find a place to sprout. When someone is diagnosed with breast cancer or lung cancer or even ovarian cancer, those types of cancer have distinct characteristics, and even if they biopsy a tumor that showed up in the lungs, it may show that it is breast cancer. Then, sure enough, they find the primary tumor in the breast and can treat it as such. With cancer of unknown primary, there isn't a primary tumor. The cancer cells start invading the healthy cells, and it kind of snowballs. The larger the cancer gets, the faster it spreads by traveling through the bloodstream and eventually taking root in various parts of the body where it begins to develop into tumors."

In Annette's case, it settled in her lungs, where by now she had hundreds of nodules growing, two tumors in her breasts, and one below her right breast. There was a large mass on her chest wall, and if that wasn't enough, the cancer invaded her spine—her first lower lumbar vertebrae, to be exact.

Then the doctor went on to say that there is no cure, and only a 10 percent chance of putting it into remission. The best that we can do is treat the symptoms and make you as comfortable as possible.

By this time I was in mild shock. I couldn't believe that things could have gotten worse, but they were, and that still wasn't the end. He continued on to say that not only are we not going to treat your cancer, but we are going to keep you here for a few days until we get your blood thin enough that you can travel without the possibility of creating a blood clot that could give you a stroke or even kill you.

We later learned that Annette carried a genetic trait called Factor 5. Factor 5 has always been around, but the doctors and researchers didn't understand it until about ten years ago when researchers tied it to genetics. Factor 5 is a clotting disorder. It causes the body to create blood clots at an accelerated rate under certain circumstances. If any good comes from Annette's disease, it will be the awareness that her family carries this disease, and they can be tested for it. The knowledge that you have the disease means that the doctors can anticipate problems during pregnancy or surgery. It's like knowing that you have an enlarged heart or clogged arteries before getting on the treadmill for a stress test. It can make a difference between life and death.

Getting back to the cancer, this is a very aggressive cancer and it spreads quickly. I can't understand—if it is such an aggressive cancer, why aren't we running to get treatment? Why are we just sitting here? We're so concerned about blood clots, we're forgetting the fact that the cancer is growing exponentially. We are at one of the best hospitals in the nation—why can't we start chemo or radiation while we are here and finish up at a hospital or cancer center closer to home when Annette is ready to travel? People live for years with cancer. I'm sure some of them move to different towns, if not states. They must have their records transferred so they can continue with treatment. I don't understand why we're just sitting here. If you remember, the doctor that came on Saturday said, and I quote, "If she's going to have any chance at all she needs to start treatment immediately." Why the contradiction? Either she needs to be treated now or not.

Sam is starting to get wound up; you could look at him and see the wheels turning. With an intense glare in his eyes, he fires question after question to the doctor as he tries to put some logical explanation to this whole mess. All the while Annette has fallen off to sleep just as a tired infant will do in the midst of a busy New York intersection.

After an intense drilling that any homicide detective would be proud of, the doctor finally stands up and says, "All of you have understand, aggressive cancers such as Annette's may spread quickly, but they also respond quickly to treatment. You need to be patient, let us get her stable before she gets pounded with chemo."

Searching for any root that may be exposed along the side of the cliff that we are now sliding out of control down, we grab hold of that morsel of hope and use it over the next five days to build a ledge that we can firmly stand on so we can start planning a strategy for Annette's recovery. With that, he wishes us well and says he will be by tomorrow to check on Annette.

What we didn't know and what the doctor didn't tell us was that this form of cancer doesn't have any specific treatment. The oncologist will give it his best shot as to which chemo treatment to go with. It's a shot in the dark, and you, more than likely, only get one shot.

At first, when I realized that the doctor held back this information, I was mad. But then I realized he was just trying to spare us any more bad news. As time passed, Dr. Mathews played a very important role in Annette's treatment. We were lucky to have him on our team. In the end, I realized how right he was about being treated closer to home. I can't tell you how many late-night trips we made to the hospital due to complications. Complications that came in the form of dehydration, high fever, uncontrollable vomiting, or indescribable pain.

Do you remember me talking about the time phenomenon? Well, this is where it is in full gear. We would spend the next five days one minute at a time. As each minute passed, that cloud of hopelessness lingered in the not-so-far-away horizon. Pulling together, each of us relying on the other for love and support, we spent the time talking about everything under the sun. We even managed to laugh once or twice. Once or twice. Out of an entire week we laughed once or twice, and we cherished that moment as you would cherish your wedding day. Think about how many times you laugh in one day. Can you remember what you laughed about yesterday? Most people can't, because it is such a frequent occurrence. Prior to this our life was filled with laughter, and yet that week we treasured the two times we were able to dismiss the agony.

As I said, Annette and I talked about everything. Of those Conversations, the hardest thing was putting together a letter to our boys from Annette. Can you imagine trying to put together a letter of love and hope while you lie in a hospital bed getting a little closer to death as each minute passed? With every word, the realization hits you that the sole reason that you are writing this letter is that it is very possible that you may not be around for their next birthday. When we talk of suffering, you automatically think of physical pain. For us, it wasn't the physical pain—even though it was quite intense, we could control it with medication. The suffering came in the form of mental and emotional trauma. To have to write a letter knowing that you won't be there to reassure your nervous son as he prepared for his first date or be part of the audience when they graduate college. Not to be there to dance with them on their wedding day or hold your grandchildren minutes after being born. To lie there in a hospital bed knowing that one month earlier you were a healthy forty-year-old mom. And that the last thing you did with your kids was take them trick-or-treating on Halloween, and today you are trying to draft a letter that expresses a lifetime of love in a few short pages. There is nothing more painful; this is the emotional abyss. The depression, the feeling of total and complete helplessness. This is the reality of terminal cancer. After a while, Annette couldn't do it anymore, and she asked me to finish the letter for her. To this day, I can't imagine the agony writing that letter must have caused her.

As she requested, I will give it to them on the day that they graduate high school. I pray that I am strong enough to console them as they read their mom's thoughts, and I pray they find comfort in her loving words of encouragement.

It was only a little over a month ago that we were making vacation plans, discussing how to remodel the main bathroom, taking care of the boys and the house, anticipating the company Christmas party, and looking forward to a Disney cruise in December. How is it that our life could change so drastically in such a short period of time?

Annette was always in shape. She never spent a great deal of money on clothes, makeup, or manicures, and she always looked great. Beautiful . . . big brown eyes with wavy brown hair. She stood five feet tall with ten feet of spirit. And she loved me. With all my faults and idiosyncrasies, she loved me. The love we shared was the Hope diamond of romance. There wasn't a minute that went by that we didn't make love to each other. Whether a gentle hug or a light shoulder massage, a glance across the room or pat on the behind, we may as well have been romping in the bed, because it carried the same excitement and sensation as physical love. Yet, here we are in such a short period of time grasping at everything and anything that will give us a glimpse of hope. Has this affected the love we have for each other? Yes, absolutely! Catastrophes of this magnitude either destroy or fortify the bonds of marriage. You wouldn't think it was possible, but it has strengthened our love. After twenty years of looking into those big brown eyes I can feel the comfort of Annette's love engulf my soul and bring peace to my heart, knowing that she loves me!

Do you remember John, our friend from Chicago? Well, I received a call from his wife, Tammy. She told me that she would be coming in on the train from Chicago to spend a couple days with Annette. The train station was just down the street from Kensington Hospital. So I told Tammy I would pick her up from the station. Naturally, the train was late (I was always under the assumption that you could set your watch by a train schedule—I guess that's only true at Petticoat Junction), but it didn't matter; there wasn't anything going on at the hospital. Besides, it gave me a chance to get out of the room and get some fresh air.

At least, I didn't think it would matter. As it turned out, there was a group of first graders there waiting to get on the train to go on a field trip. All it did was remind me of Annette; this is exactly where she would be if it was one of our boys going on that field trip. I began to cry . . . not sobbing, but the tears were rolling down my cheek.

That's when a little girl came up and asked, "Why are you crying?"
I told her that my wife was very sick and that makes me sad.
She left briefly only to return, looking up at me with the innocence that only a six-year-old could have. Her tiny voice said, "My mommy gives me a cookie when I feel sad," as she raised her tiny hand offering the last half of her cookie to me.

I graciously turned down the cookie, but it did make me smile. The excitement in the station began to rise as all of the children could see the train pulling into the station. Looking down the track, I could see Tammy stepping off and heading toward the station. As I walked toward her, I could see her cheerful smile begin to fade away as she looked into my eyes. I sensed she could feel the anguish that was so visibly displayed on my face. She dropped her bag and embraced me with a hug that was full of love—the same kind of hug that you would extend to a child that has taken a bad fall or badly skinned a knee.

Each day was a reminder of everything that may no longer be. The day before Tammy came, Annette's sister Angie came to the hospital to give me a break and visit with Annette. So I took advantage of the time and went off to Meijers, a local store, to buy Christmas gifts for the boys. This was always something Annette and I did together. I found myself lost and in a quandary as to what should I buy. I didn't know sizes. I couldn't remember which kid liked what style. I knew Zachary needed a new fishing reel, but I couldn't even remember what style rod he had. It was so painful thinking that this may be my life. I may never go Christmas shopping, or any shopping, for that matter, with Annette again.

Tammy's mother had cancer a year or two before, and she beat the cancer, but her heart gave out, and she died shortly after completing treatment. When Tammy arrived, I told her that it was very likely that we would be going home the next day. Rather than cutting this trip short, Tammy said she would come home with us. The next few days were going to be busy, so Tammy offered to be available for the boys while I took Annette to see the oncologist. The boys got along well with Tammy and I knew she could handle their schedules. Tammy is pretty easy to talk to, or should I say listen to. I kid her because sometimes she gets rolling and you can hardly get a word in. After putting Annette to bed, we would talk about what she went through with her mother. The nice thing about talking to Tammy was she didn't barrage me with questions about Annette. Tammy understood that after I put Annette to bed, it was my time to download. All day long my time was spent dealing with Annette and all the issues that came with her illness. This time of night was my time to escape and just vegetate.

On the second night we started talking about some of the decisions her and her mother had to make, one of which was treatment. Do you pursue treatment or not? The possibility that it may be in Annette's best interests not to pursue treatment was horrifying to me. I didn't like being put in that position. I just spent weeks being faced with what facility or doctor should I take her to, and now I'm being told that I have to decide on whether to fight for her life or let her go. That thought was beyond comprehension at this point in the game. Later I learned that this same question would rear its ugly head once again. But, for now, that's not an option. I expressed that to Tammy, and she backed off.

As difficult or as unimaginable as it may be, some cancer patients are at a stage that treatment may not help. All that ends up happening is the little time they have left is spent miserably from the side effects of chemo. Even though Annette was only forty, it may still become a reality that this may be all the time she has. As hard as it is to accept; it is a fact that people do die young. Unfortunately, life does not have a time quota. Children die, babies die, and Annette could die. At this moment in time, life STINKS!

The day we were to leave Kensington Hospital I was running around the hospital gathering up CAT scans, X-rays, and reports. I ran into a young mother and her baby who had become lost in the maze of hallways below Kensington Hospital, so I offered to show her the way back to the elevators. Along the way, we talked and she told me that her daughter was diagnosed with Crohn's disease.

Just as we reached the elevator, she asked, "What is wrong with your wife?"

I responded, "She has cancer." I left it at that.

As she was stepping onto the elevator she said, "At least your wife has something that can be cured. My daughter is only expected to live for a couple more years."

I didn't respond other than to wish her well and that God be with her. As I walked to my elevator, I realized that I needed to deal with this situation in a brighter light. As difficult as that may seem, I needed to savor every moment that we had left and not become consumed that Annette will die and, more than likely, die soon. I hope that young mother realizes that she needs to live every day with as bright of an outlook as possible and not dwell on the end; it will come soon enough.

Annette and I never anticipated the end of whatever we were doing. For example, you're on vacation and you're talking to another couple, and one of them says, "We only have six days left of our seven-day vacation." These people are living for the end. Why not view it as "We have only been here for one day, and we have six more wonderful days left"?

Hopes and Fears

The next day, we left the hospital. At first I thought we were going straight from Kensington Hospital to the cancer-treatment center, but I was wrong. Cancer treatment is an outpatient procedure. All appointments and treatment times have to be scheduled in advance. So we went home and called. At first the receptionist started to tell me that the earliest opening was fifteen days away. FIFTEEN DAYS? What the heck was going on here? For the last week we had been told that immediate treatment is required if Annette is going to have any chance at all. How can everyone we talk to be so casual about this? We are in a race for survival, and the ambulance driver is taking the scenic route.

That's when all of my sales experience kicked in. I never liked the label "sales"; to me, it carried an undertone of distrust. However, this was war and, as they say. "all's fair." I had the name of the doctor we were to see, but that's all I had. Starting off calmly, I quickly began to increase the intensity in my tone. I'm not saying the receptionist was giving me a hard time; in fact, she was very much in our corner. I just wasn't going to give her any room to sway. I started making up a story of how we were scheduled to see the doctor today, but their office dropped the ball and didn't get it on the appointment schedule. I told her Dr. Mathews at Kensington Hospital personally called and talked to Dr. Kimpali, and we were supposed to come in TODAY! I'm not waiting 2 weeks . . .

We had an appointment for the next day.

We had been at Kensington Hospital for seven days. Seven days we waited to get released so we could go to a different location to treat the cancer that was consuming Annette's body at an accelerated rate. The cancer was growing at an exponential rate; we didn't have time to wait. We needed to start treatment as quickly as possible, and they knew it. Do you think, I repeat, DO YOU THINK someone at Kensington Hospital would have come to us the first day and said, "Here, take this card . . . this is who you need to call" or "Here is the name of a doctor that we recommend you see . . . call them now, and make an appointment for around a week from now"? If you ever find yourself in this position, find an organizer. Find someone who is close enough to care but far enough removed to think clearly. You need someone that can run scenarios and try to anticipate what would be needed next. That was always my job. I was the idea guy, and Annette put everything into motion. Annette obviously couldn't participate, and my mind was mush. By this time, I had a hard time remembering what I ordered at the fast-food counter. So find someone that can fill this need. It is very crucial to keep as much emotional stress as you can to a minimum. Organization and planning always keep stress to a minimum.

December 13, 2002—the day we started the next leg of the marathon. I didn't even realize that it was Friday, the 13th. We had an appointment to see Dr. Kimpali, and I asked Sam to join us. As with all the other times that we moved to a different facility or when we met with a different person, they wanted to know how this all began. After telling Annette's story, Dr. Kimpali turned to Annette and said,

"My sister (Dr. Kimpali is from Africa, and he has a very interesting accent), I'm so very sorry. I will do the best I can, but I cannot lie to you. The treatment that you have to endure is very harsh, and it is possible that you may die from the treatment itself."

Another blow. Is there anything about this, that's going to be somewhat easy? It just seems that every time we turn around someone is reminding us that Annette has the worst of the worst cancer.

At this point, Annette can barely sit up. She is so medicated I'm surprised she's even conscious. When the doctor stops talking, she slowly lifts her head and says, "There is a tumor under my right breast."

Dr. Kimpali jumps to his feet and asks, "Can I please see this? If you don't mind, I would like to examine you."

Why do doctors ask this question, Do you mind if I examine you? One of these times I'm going to say, "YES, I do mind! Go stand on the other side of the room, and give us your best diagnosis from there." I figure some doctor somewhere was sued by some nutcase for touching them before asking permission. I mean, what the heck do you think we are here for?

YES, please! Examine her wherever you feel you have to. It just amazes me.

After examining Annette, Dr. Kimpali abruptly leaves the room. He returned shortly and said he was trying to get Annette in to see the surgeon for a biopsy and get an ultrasound of her breast. It was then that I asked him if he was aware that one of the stains from the original biopsy came back along the germ cell line. His eyes lit up, and he ran out of the room again. Annette was scheduled for an ultrasound. We had scheduled it the Friday before. It was one of the things Doctor Kimpali wanted done before deciding on which treatment to start Annette on. While the doctor was gone, Sam left with Annette and headed to X-ray. When Dr. Kimpali returned, he said, "I just scheduled Annette for a CAT scan, and I would like to hold off on starting treatment until the results come in."

HOLD OFF ON TREATMENT!? What did I do?

We were in reach of starting treatment. We were there, and I just delayed it for another week or two. I couldn't believe it. STUPID, STUPID, STUPID. What a dope. I can tell you, It hurts to think sometimes.

There wasn't any time to think about it, though. Sam had already taken Annette to have the ultrasound done. When I caught up with them, I told Annette that Dr. Kimpali wanted to postpone treatment until the results of the CAT scan came in. She was upset with me—I mean, downright pissed off. Then her big brown eyes began to tear up. "I can't wait any longer to start treatment. I'll die before they make up their minds as to what to do."

She wasn't saying anything that the rest of us weren't already thinking. Just then, the nurse came and wheeled Annette in for her test.

Not able to sit down, I was pacing back and forth. I never felt panic before now. My mind was racing. Somehow I had to undo what I just did, so I went back down the hall to Dr. Kimpali's office to put Annette back on the schedule to start treatment Monday.

I was only gone maybe fifteen minutes, but when I returned, they were closed. One o'clock in the afternoon, and they were closed. Just our luck we would have an appointment on the day of their Christmas party. See why I don't rely on luck? Luck stinks! Oh, by the way, it was Friday, so you know what that means. They're closed until Monday.

The tension was overwhelming, and the stress of having to wait until Monday just to talk to the doctor about waiting on treatment would have been too much. Just by chance, Dr. Kimpali called me on my cell phone. I told him that Annette was devastated about the postponement of treatment. I also explained to him that I couldn't get in for the CAT scan until the end of the next week. This meant that because Annette's treatment had to go five days in a row and because the week after her CAT scan was Christmas week and the following week was New Year's (both are partial workweeks), she wouldn't be able to start treatment for a month. Dr. Kimpali didn't realize this and said he would look into speeding things up. I felt pretty good, and even though I wasn't promised anything, I told Annette that I talked to the doctor, and he would keep her treatment as scheduled. She started crying again, but this time it was out of relief, not grief.

Nothing was carved into stone yet for Monday, but it wouldn't have done her any good to worry about it. Before leaving the surgeon's office, the doctor came in and explained that the growth didn't feel like a tumor, but it didn't feel like a cist either.

It was believed that the growth under Annette's breast was a key factor in reaching a firm conclusion as to what had invaded her body, so we went ahead and scheduled to have it removed on Monday. Until then, it was anybody's guess as to what it actually was.

By the way, do you remember when I told you about the exam Annette received at Kensington Hospital by the "gray hair," the guy that dropped in on Saturday morning and gave his diagnosis? The same person that sent us all into the depth of anguish and despair when he announced that

Annette had not two tumors but twelve tumors in her breasts? According to that doctor, ten more tumors had appeared in her breasts in just one day. Well, the surgeon explained to Annette and me that these were everyday cists, not tumors—the same cists that are found in most women over forty. If I wasn't so relieved at the news I would have called Kensington Hospital on the spot and told them what I thought of their "prominent doctor." There is a reason some corporations have a mandatory retirement policy. What a Jerk – that's jerk with a capitol J- to give that kind of news to a patient without any proof.

We went home that night feeling really good. After spending six weeks spinning our tires in an endless mud pit, we were actually on the road and picking up speed.

That night our spirits were high; we felt we could beat this thing. The boys were at Bill and Angie's house for the weekend, so it would be quiet and calm at home. When we made it home, I got Annette settled in and started a bath for her. Because she lost so much weight, she would get cold very easily. In an effort to keep her as comfortable as possible, I removed the register from the bathroom heat duct, turned up the thermostat, and ran a tub of water. It didn't take long before the bathroom was like a sauna.

With the blood clot still in her arterial vein going to her lungs, Annette was on oxygen and didn't have the strength to walk, so I carried her up to the bathroom. Once there, I quickly undressed her and helped her into the tub. Even with the register off and the heat turned up, it didn't take long for Annette to get cold. Besides, it took a lot of energy, energy she didn't have just to sit there. Memories of the times we shared bathing together would remind me of the passion we shared. I may have wanted to savor the moment and make every pass of the washcloth last as long as possible, but Annette was doing everything she could to keep sitting in an upright position, so I hurried along as quickly as I could. After the bath, I dressed her and carried her to bed.

Before Annette became ill, it wasn't unusual for us to light a candle and lie in bed and talk, so tonight, for the first time in months, I lit her favorite candle, turned out the lights, and held her close to me as she drifted off to sleep. That night as she drifted off, I leaned over to kiss her and tell her good night. That's when Annette opened one eye and said, "Would you like a little action?"

"You're kidding, right?"

"No," she said with a devilish grin. "Come here."

"Really?" I replied.

"Yes. Come on."

As I leaned closer, she raised her head, kissed my cheek, and fell asleep. It was the first night in a month that we both slept the entire night peacefully. There's nothing like a wild session to relieve the day's stress.

The next day, Saturday, December 14 about eight thirty, I received a call from Dr. Kimpali at home. Yeah, that's right, at eight thirty in the evening—a Saturday evening on top of it—I get a call from Annette's doctor. He wants to see us Monday morning at eight. He is going to start her treatment and wants to do another exam before starting. There were tears in my eyes when I hung up the phone. Not just about the fact that Annette was going to start receiving chemo on Monday, but she had a doctor that cared enough to call her personally on a Saturday night, not only to check on her but to give me his home phone number in case we needed him.

Monday morning came, and Dr. Kimpali explained to Annette that he was going to treat her along the germ cell line. Germ cell cancers are very treatable, even curable. Once again, our souls had been lifted. We couldn't believe what we were hearing. Just last week at Kensington Hospital we were told that Annette's chances of survival were very grim. In their defense, the results of the germ cell slide stain hadn't come in while we were there.

If you haven't caught on by now, when you are dealing with cancer, it's kind of like the weather in Michigan: give it an hour, and you'll be looking at a whole new day. The one thing that you can bet on is that if you wait long enough, things will change, and you will find that you're heading down another road. Unless you have what I call a mainline cancer, such as breast or lung cancer, where the treatment is very defined and you have a multitude of treatments at hand to try, your experience will be one of uncertainty. (Please know that I'm not diminishing the seriousness of these forms of cancer. They are very deadly and can be just as devastating to the families involved. It's just a fact that these cancers are curable, and the chance of survival is much greater than a diagnosis of an unknown primary type of cancer.) One day you're up, the next day you're down, and I'm not talking about how she feels—I'm talking about survival. One day you're on the road to recovery; the next day you have a bad reaction to the treatment, and the medical community begins to have doubt.

That Monday we arrived at the Cancer Treatment Center. The treatment center is an interesting facility. It is designed to give you a very warm feeling the minute you come through the doors. There is a great deal of cherry wood and hardwood flooring, with carpeting down the main aisleway. The ladies at the front desk address you by name on your first visit, as if you have been there many times before. The treatment area itself is a long area with reclining chairs, one after the other. Each chair can be closed off with curtains, much like in an emergency room. There is a TV between every two chairs, along with a small cupboard, which contains pillows and blankets that the patients can use. (There is something about chemo treatments that seems to make people cold.) They have a patient pantry where you can get a cup of coffee, tea, or hot chocolate, along with a small refrigerator that has a wide variety of juices to choose from. There is even a microwave to warm up something for lunch. That is a nice feature for those of us that spend six to eight hours there every time we come in. There is also a selection of cakes and crackers set out to snack on—all at no charge. My point is they seem to try and make you feel as comfortable as they can. It has to be hard to work here. Yes, they have their successes, but they have those who they don't save, and from what I can tell, it doesn't stop them from getting close to their patients. These people have strong spirits and huge hearts.

When Annette started her treatment, she had a hard time with even the more tolerable drugs. She ran into so many complications the first morning that we weren't able to complete that day's treatment before she had to leave for the lumpectomy. I was very concerned. The lump wasn't going anywhere; we could do it another day. I wanted to stay and continue on with the chemo, but they said the surgery shouldn't take long, and Annette could come back and finish the chemo in the afternoon.

The frustration and concern began to mount as Annette's surgery was delayed because of her reaction to the morning chemo. I guess it threw things out of whack, and they needed to let her body adjust before they began surgery. By the time Annette was able to have the lump removed, she had missed her scheduled time and now had to wait for a break in the schedule. It was almost three thirty before they wheeled her in; we had left for the surgery at eleven thirty. There was no chance of completing Annette's treatment today. Besides, she was exhausted and sore from the chemo and the surgery. It was a long day; we left the house at seven that morning, and it was close to five o'clock when she came out of recovery, so I wheeled her out to the car and took her home.

We seemed to be moving so quickly now, yet it felt as though we weren't accomplishing anything. It reminded me of my time in the service. You get orders to hurry up and go somewhere just so you could turn around and come back. We continued that week to try and get all of the chemo into Annette, but every day presented another problem. By the end of the week, Annette managed to receive about 75 percent of the treatment. I wasn't very happy, but the nurses told me that this is a very brutal regimen, and it is common for a patient to have complications and not to worry about it. Five days straight of chemotherapy is very hard on the body, and considering that Annette was extremely weak, it was a miracle that she tolerated as much as she did.

The weekend brought even more misery. Just because Annette didn't receive her full dose of chemo didn't mean she was off the hook for the full dose of side effects. All weekend long she just couldn't stop throwing up. When I say throwing up, I'm not talking about the same kind of thing that happens when you get sick. When you are sick with an upset stomach, once your stomach is empty, the nausea generally stops. These side effects, however, don't. My poor angel continued to have dry heaves all weekend. Once in a while, she would be able to get down some fluids and maybe a little food, but that usually came with total retaliation from her body. It was a vicious circle: Annette would throw up until she literally passed out. After a short rest, we would try and get some nourishment into her, but this only provoked her body into a brutal frenzy. Finally, we gave up trying to feed her. I had Annette slowly sip water; if nothing else, I had to try and keep her hydrated.

The Christmas Present

Bill was over on Monday, December 23rd, to see how Annette was doing. I told him she wasn't eating much, and she was much weaker. He told us that the doctors may admit her to receive nourishment and get rehydrated, so the next morning we left for her appointment, anticipating having to go to the hospital.

The next day, Tuesday, December 24th, Christmas Eve, Annette was scheduled to receive her Bleomyacin treatment, but she was in no condition to be poisoned again. That's what chemo is—it's poison. They shoot it into your veins, and it travels through your body attacking the cancer cells, killing them off. The problem is, it doesn't stop with the cancer cells. It also attacks the healthy cells. Chemotherapy cannot distinguish between cancer cells and healthy cells; it destroys everything in its path. If I understand this correctly, cancerous blood cells are the food that feed the tumors, and the idea behind chemotherapy is to remove the food supply to the tumors by killing off the cancerous cells. Yes, the treatment will kill off good, healthy cells in the process, but we rely on the body to produce enough healthy cells to replace both the cancerous cells and the healthy cells that are lost in the battle.

I remember a story from the Bible. (I'm sure this won't be completely accurate, but you will get the idea.) The story goes like this: Jesus is standing outside a city that has become invaded by evil and immorality. He tells his disciple that he is going to punish the people that have turned away from God's teaching by destroying the city.

His disciple speaks up and says, "Lord, if I can find one hundred faithful people, will you spare the city?"
"Yes," Jesus replies.
Then the disciple asks again. "Lord, if I can find fifty people, will you spare the city?"
"Yes," Jesus replies.
Once again, the disciple asks, "Lord, if I can find twenty or even ten people, will you spare the city?"

And, again, Jesus accepts the offer to spare the city if he can find ten good people.

Then, in a bold move, the disciple asks, "Lord, if I can find one person, will you spare the city?"

"Yes, I will spare the city."

The point I'm trying to make is that it only takes one person, one individual with the conviction to stand alone and present to the others that there is always hope, that there is always a light at the end of the tunnel. Have faith, and support those who are willing to work toward healing the body and conquering the evil invader. I'm not sure why I think this applies to Annette's cancer; it just seems as though the cancerous cells represent the evil and immorality, and the healthy cells represent the good and faithful. The healthy cells are standing strong against the evil cells. Unfortunately, the healthy cells cannot resist the overwhelming force of the evil cancerous cells. To add to this, our only defense against the evil cancerous cells is a method that wipes out the innocent healthy cells in the process. Much like the solution that Jesus was presenting, wipe out the entire city as a means of conquering the evil. Now I'm sure there is a much deeper meaning to the story, however this is all I need to make my point.

I ask you to support those at St. Jude Children's Research Hospital and the American Cancer Society. These are the people with the conviction to stand up and say "there must be a better way". The miracle for cancer patients is the discovery of a treatment that will only attack the cancerous cells, leaving the healthy cells to heal the body. Jesus' disciple was the miracle cure for the city; he gathered his conviction and courage to question his Lord's intent. He brought to the table the fact that there is always another option; you just have to be willing to look for it.

Getting back to Tuesday, the 24th, just as Bill had said, Dr. Kimpali had decided to admit Annette into the hospital to build up her vitals and blood counts. What I wasn't prepared for was what happened next.

While we were still at the cancer center waiting for the nurse to come back with the results of Annette's blood work, Rita came to the doorway and motioned me to follow her. Annette was sleeping, so I snuggled Annette's blanket around her and walked toward Rita. Tucking her hand on the cuff of my arm, she walked with me down the hall to an examination room. She set me in a chair and told me that Dr. Kimpali wanted to talk to me. I didn't realize I was going for a private consult. Rita is one of the veteran nurses. She is constantly being asked by some of the other nurses to help with this thing or that thing, and they regularly come to her to get her opinion. Being asked to wait in one of the examining rooms didn't surprise me as much as the fact that Rita was staying with me. This put a rock in my stomach. Dr. Kimpali came in and sat down beside me.

He started out with, "I'm very sorry. I pray for you and Annette. I have received the results of the lumpectomy. The biopsy had showed that the cancer is a sarcoma, and it is in the fourth stage."

I'm not sure what a sarcoma is, but unlike a germ cell cancer, it isn't curable, and it is very difficult to put into remission. This is one of those times where the outlook of the patient is a vital part of the treatment. If the patient loses faith and begins to get discouraged, they don't stand a chance of beating the cancer. The patient has to believe that they are going to be alright and have a strong desire to survive in order for the treatment to be effective.

At the time, I didn't realize that Annette's cancer was already in the fourth stage. There are no more stages; that's the end of the line. Fourth-stage cancer means the tumor has spread to the lymph nodes and or other parts of the body such as lungs, breasts, liver, bones, and any other part of the body that blood flows to. I knew Annette's cancer had spread; I didn't realize it was considered fourth stage or metastasized. Fourth-stage or metastasized cancer is the end of the line. Not that there isn't any hope; there just isn't much rope left to hold onto . . . a dim situation, at best.

I was just sitting there with my mind wondering aimlessly when Dr. Kimpali touches my arm and says, "My brother, I'm very sorry." He hesitates, wipes his eyes, and says, "You know, Annette is my age, and I'm very sorry."

I could see the pain in his eyes. Then I looked to Rita, and she had a tear running down her face. These people deal with this every single day, and it still hits hard when they see someone so young and healthy be attacked so viscously. I didn't want to, but I knew I had to ask how long. How much longer did I have left to look at her beautiful face? How many more times would I feel her lips kiss mine? When you are talking about how much longer your forty-year-old wife has to live, the words just don't come. It's not conceivable. It hangs out there just out of reach. You know it is there, but it just doesn't seem real.

After what seems like an eternity, Dr. Kimpali asks, "Does she have a strong desire to live, or has she begun to give in to the pain and suffering? I may be able to put it into remission if she is willing to fight, but she has to keep a very positive outlook, or she won't make it."

With my head down resting in my hands, I ask, "How long?"

Dr. Kimpali replies, "If we can't put it into remission, maybe two months."

I must have been in shock, because I didn't even flinch. I sat there looking at him and then at Rita. I couldn't cry; I didn't yell or hit anything. I just sat there.

After what seemed like an hour, I ask, "When you say remission, what does that mean? Will Annette live a normal life as she did before? Would it be semi-normal where she will be in and out of the hospital receiving treatment, and for how long?"

With a slight pause, Dr. Kimpali says, "In Annette's case, remission means keeping her alive for maybe one or two, possibly three, years on the outside."

Alive, yes. Living, no! Chances are, she would be bedridden. She would spend most of her time heavily sedated to keep the pain under control. She wouldn't be able to travel or face off an opponent at a seven-card stud table in Las Vegas or feel the thrill of the latest roller coaster at Cedar Point. Going on a cruise would be out of the question, as would simply enjoying a quiet, romantic evening in bed. Annette would be breathing, but she wouldn't be living the life she cherished so deeply.

When we were at Kensington Hospital, they talked about not being able to cure her. Dr. Mathews said the best they could do would be to treat the symptoms to relieve the pain. At that time, I didn't ask how long. I couldn't. It was easier to assume that it would take years before the cancer would win. In my mind, I began to believe it. I didn't need someone to verify it for me. I just knew she wouldn't leave me anytime soon. I was faced with the very thing that Tammy tried to bring to light a couple of weeks ago. I was devastated. The horror of reality was upon me. Annette was going to die.

After a brief moment I left the room, squeezing Rita's hand as I walked past. Annette was still sleeping, so I whispered softly to her "honey wake up, Dr Kimpali wants you to check into the hospital" she gently nodded. After gathering up her things we headed back to the car. That was the saddest walk I ever made.

I didn't tell anyone what the doctor had told me. It was Christmas Eve—how could I tell her family that Annette only had a very short time left on this earth?

I had invited Mike, Kim, and the girls to spend Christmas Eve night with us. Their house was still being rebuilt from the fire that they had. Did I tell you? They had the fire the same night we found out Annette had cancer. I couldn't see them spending Christmas in a hotel room. We get along so well, I thought it would be nice for everyone to spend Christmas morning together.

After a busy morning of opening gifts and getting breakfast for seven kids and three adults, we all managed to get dressed to head for the hospital to see Annette. It had snowed that night. We had clear skies and about four inches of fresh snow. It was a bright day; the sun was glistening off the snow. Annette had a window next to her bed with a nice view. The boys were very excited to see her. We brought a few gifts with us for Annette to open. I took pictures and played Christmas music on the CD player. Each of the boys took turns lying in bed with their mom. They shared hugs and kisses and talked about the gifts they had gotten. They missed her; it seemed every time she went to the doctor for a test or exam, she didn't come home for a week. We had all the makings for a wonderful Christmas. The spirit of Christmas prevailed, despite our situation and the location of our celebration.

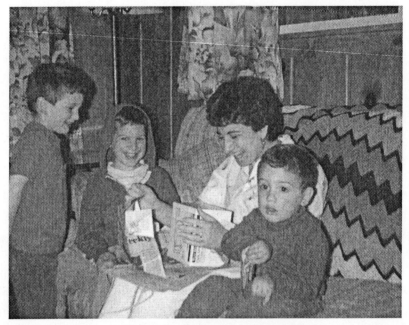

Christmas 1995 at Houghton Lake.

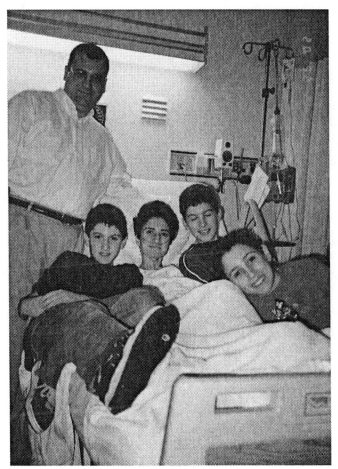

Christmas morning, 2003

After a few hours, Annette was very tired, so the boys and I and our friends said, "See you later." (In our home, we never say "good-bye.") We headed off to Bill and Angie's house for dinner. Still keeping my secret, I was in no mood for company. It took all I had to keep it inside that morning.

Once I said my hellos, I told Bill I needed to get some sleep. Although I did fall asleep, the real reason I slipped away was the fact that I just couldn't face anyone. I just wanted to be alone. I knew that sooner or later they would want to start asking questions about what the doctor said. Everyone knew we had gone to the doctor the day before, only this time I didn't call them and fill in all of the details like I did in the past.

Around five o'clock I couldn't avoid it any longer. It was time to eat dinner, and someone came up to wake me. I had been awake for a while; I was sitting there staring out the window crying. Not wanting to be seen crying, I turned away as they stuck their head in the door to call me. As the door opened, I immediately said "I heard" and that I would be down shortly. When they left I went to the bathroom to wash my face so as to not to appear that anything was wrong. When dinner was finished and the dishes were cleared, I went to the living room and sat with the kids, watching them play with their new games. First, Sam came in, and then Joann. They started off slowly with an occasional question, then Lisa came in with her questions. At first I tried to avoid any in-depth answer, dancing around question after question, but the more I danced, the more suspicious they became, and I could see they weren't going to let up. So I sent all the kids downstairs and gathered all the adults in the kitchen. I told Bill, who at the time was standing at the sink doing dishes, to jump in if I left out anything.

I couldn't say it. I couldn't get out even one syllable, and I was avoiding making eye contact. The longer it took to start, the more anxious they all became. I couldn't help it; every time I started to tell them my secret, I started to break down. Finally, Bill came and stood next to me, put his arm over my shoulder and said, "Go ahead. We're all here with you."

Taking a deep breath to gain my composure, I started with, "Annette's biopsy of the lump in her breast came back. It's what they call a sarcoma."

"Well, what does that mean?" Lisa asks.

"It means there isn't a cure," I replied.

"What does that mean?" Lisa asked. "Can't they stop it from growing?" she asks again.

I can hear the panic building in her voice, and as I look around the room, I can see the pain in their eyes and the tears running down their faces as everyone begins to feel that elusive demon burrow into their being.

As Bill holds me closer, he encourages me on. "Go on, Roc," he says.

Clinching Bill's hand in mine, I stumble over the words. "It means Annette isn't going to make it. Dr. Kimpali said that in all likeliness Annette only has a couple more months."

I don't have to tell what happened next. Some Christmas present. Every time I think of that moment I get a lump in my throat, and my eyes well up with tears.

Annette would spend the next week in the hospital. I spent the days reading to her, whether it was all of the get-well cards she received or her daily prayer booklet. It didn't matter. All we wanted was to communicate with each other. I wanted to hear her voice as often as I could, and I wanted her to hear mine. When you are experiencing the kind of tragedy we were, there is a great deal of comfort when you hear the voice of the one you love. I would rub her back and legs, trying to keep the blood circulating to avoid bed sores. I helped her eat and gave her sponge baths. After every bath I would rub her down with lotion; we both came to enjoy that part. We also spent time comforting each other's emotions. Most of all, we began to cherish every moment we had.

Of the many friends that came to visit Annette; we had one visitor we could have done without. She was there for a follow-up test. She had breast cancer, and she needed to have a test done to see if the cancer was still in remission. When she walked in, she put her coat down and said to Annette, and I quote, "Cancer is such an inconvenience. I was supposed to get my hair done today, but this was the only time they could see me."

You witch, I thought to myself. Annette is dying, and she's complaining to Annette because her hair appointment got screwed up. I was so upset I was going to say something, but Annette's mom grabbed my arm and shook her head.

"It's OK." she said, almost without a sound, and then she flipped her head toward Annette.

I looked at Annette and she gave me the look. I knew that look. It was the "let it go, it's not that important" look, so I did. Annette conveniently fell asleep within a few minutes.

Now you would think the visitor would get the message and leave. No. She starts up a conversation with the lady in the next bed—not a quiet conversation either. Finally, I told her that Annette needed her rest. Her response was, "That's OK. I'll visit with this lady."

"No!" I said. "Annette needs her rest, and she needs it to be quiet."

"Oh," she says. "Well, tell Annette I said good-bye."

"Yeah. I'll be sure to do that."

It happens more than you would think. People are so involved in their own lives that they are oblivious to everything around them. You know who gets it? Kids. Kids get it with all of the compassion of a saint. There wasn't a child that we knew that didn't send Annette a card or some type of gift to show that they were sorry she was so sick and that they hoped and prayed that she would recover.

D Day

While at the hospital this time, the pain in Annette's back was growing more severe. After another CAT scan of her back, we learned that the tumor in her back had attacked the first lower lumbar vertebrae in her spine. When this happens, the bone becomes very soft. Because of the location of the vertebrae, there is a lot of pressure on that bone, and it was beginning to fracture. This meant that Annette would have to start radiation therapy to try and beat back the tumor and allow the bone to heal. For the next ten days she would receive a dose of radiation. Radiation therapy is a very small dose of radiation pinpointed to a very specific location. As it turned out, Annette's gastrointestinal tract was right in the way. They didn't expect it to, but it caused some trouble in her digestive tract, which sparked about three weeks of constant indigestion and vomiting. She just can't catch a break.

The radiation treatment interrupted Annette's chemo cycle by one week. I thought with the break in chemo she would be stronger and healthier, making her able to tolerate the treatment more successfully this time around. But it didn't go any better. This cycle was plagued with constant nausea, the inability to eat coupled with extreme fatigue.

Annette was so weak I continued to carry her around the house. It was all she could do to get up and walk to the bathroom. On the sixteenth day of her second cycle she was so weak that I was terrified that she would die of malnutrition. Annette weighed 105 pounds when she went to the hospital on November 5. Today, she hit a whopping 76 pounds.

Annette was slowly dying, and I couldn't do anything about it.

Once again, because of her condition, she didn't receive her chemo. It would have killed her. I did convince the doctor to set up IV nutrition that I could dispense at home. It is called a TPN bag, and it has all the nutrition that she needs to keep all of her main organs functioning normally and enough calories to actually start putting weight back on her bones—all without having to eat a thing. I was so happy to have the TPN bag. You see prior to this, trying to get Annette to eat anything was frustratingly painful. Every morsel was shadowed by the thought, Is it this one that's going to trigger the vomiting? Or maybe the next one? I'm not talking about a full meal with meat and potatoes. A meal for Annette consisted of a saltine cracker and one-thirds of a cup of chicken soup. Infants eat more in one sitting. Yet each bite came with a prayer that she would be able to get it down and keep it there.

As I mentioned earlier, this combination of cancer that Annette has is very rare, and her reaction to the chemo is new territory. It seems the doctors and nurses expect to run into bad reactions and poor blood counts, but in Annette's case, the severity of the reactions is outside the norm. All this time I had been keeping track of and logging her medication. I wrote down the dose and time that I gave it to her, her weight, and if she was throwing up or not. I even kept track of if she was eating or drinking and how much. I don't know why I kept track the way I did, but I'm glad I did. After a while I gained the confidence of the doctors and nurses to the point where they didn't question what I was telling them and even, on occasion, asked my opinion if I thought a certain routine or treatment would help based on her history and reaction to other methods. Don't get me wrong. I'm not a doctor or nurse by any stretch of the imagination, but I was able to give them insight into her condition after we left the treatment center or hospital. This was information that they rarely had access to; in fact, in most cases, they have to guess as to what was going on at home between visits. My records enabled them to eliminate the guesswork.

At this point, Annette had not been able to complete an entire twenty-one-day cycle of treatment. By the time she finished the first five days of treatment, her blood count was too low, and she just wasn't in good enough health to receive any more chemo. Even with the TPN bag Annette's blood count was still dropping below treatment level.

As with all of us, Annette's physical well-being is directly related to her blood count. The lower her blood and platelet counts, the weaker she would be. Because of my relationship with the doctors and nurses, I requested that Annette get a CBC blood test four days before her next treatment. After explaining the reason for my request, they were more than happy to oblige. You see, instead of waiting for treatment day to run blood work to see if she was healthy enough (meaning, strong enough to receive chemo), I wanted to test her prior to that and get her a transfusion a couple days before so she would have a chance at being strong enough to receive chemo when the time came.

I'm not trying to blow my own horn. I included this in here so you know that you have to take an aggressive interest in the care of your loved ones. Annette has the best team of doctors and nurses that you could ask for. Even with that, they cannot focus their time on an individual basis the way you can. Don't be afraid to tell the nurse where they have the best luck drawing blood or ask what's in the bag that they are hanging on the IV pole. Learn the dosages and frequency that the drug can be given. This way, you can suggest or ask for a certain sedative or nausea medication. Knowing what the drugs are, what they are for, and how often you can give them will allow you to work with the medical team to provide the most attentive care possible.

We found that some nurses feel that you are stepping on their toes, but they will still get what you want if they can; they won't deny you. However, most nurses appreciate the help, and I haven't met a doctor yet that didn't stop and take note that you are an active participant. They know the importance of the insight that you can provide. Don't be afraid to help either. Ask for the bed linens so you can change the sheets. Most of the time, they will tell you that they will do it. Graciously decline and tell them that they have enough to worry about and that you don't mind doing it. Or take that little pitcher that they give you for water to the nurses' station instead of ringing the buzzer, and ask for ice or water. Again, they will tell you that they will bring it. Decline again, and tell them it's alright, you really don't mind. Nurses, just like anyone else, like to be appreciated. Not only do you start to make a lot of friends, but when you really need that sedative or medication, it is amazing how quickly you go to the top of the list. They also start taking a stronger interest in the care you receive. In Annette's case, when her back was at its worst from the tumors' invasion of her bone, one of the nurses tracked down a soft sheepskin swatch that she could lie on. Keep in mind that this nurse found it in another ward four floors down. Annette didn't go anywhere after that without that sheepskin. It pays to show you care.

On Saturday, March 8, Annette began throwing up blood. I called Dr. Kimpali and, not to my surprise, he asked me to bring her into the emergency room. It was another strange weather day in Michigan. All day long it was fairly mild, then just about when Annette began to get sick, it started to snow. By the time I was able to dress her and get her out to the car, the snow had turned to rain. While driving to the hospital, the temperature dropped twenty degrees, and all of the rain was beginning to freeze. I told Annette that for being the planner that she is, she sure didn't plan this well at all. To become sick in the middle of a Michigan winter was not one of her greater accomplishments. She responded with, "You just never mind. I can throw up while you drive." That comment illustrates Annette's persona to the tee. With all that she has endured, after twenty-eight treatments of chemo, three blood transfusions, and an endless barrage of needles being poked into her arm, she still had her wit. Never once did she ever feel sorry for herself or complain "Why me?" As a friend of mine put it after a visit not too long ago, "Annette truly is a beautiful person."

Today is the thirteenth of March, and we are all pleased to see that Annette has exceeded the timeframe that she was originally given at the end of December. If you remember, it was felt that she probably wouldn't make it beyond two months.

Annette was on a very rigorous treatment. The first five days of her treatment she received two drugs—one was called Cisplatin and the other Etoposide. On the second, ninth, and sixteenth day she received Bleomyacin. It seems most cancer patients receive a dose of chemo once a week or once every two weeks. They receive one treatment and then have one or two weeks to recover. Annette's regimen called for five straight days of treatment in the beginning of the cycle. That's a lot of poison! Her cycles were twenty-one days long and she had just completed the fourth cycle.

This was a critical time. This is where we learned whether the chemotherapy was working or not. A CAT scan was done after the second week, but it didn't show much of a result. The doctors felt it may have been a little premature to use it as a measurement of progress, but they had other concerns at the time. So we were hinging on the results of this next CAT scan. A great deal of hopes and prayers went into this test. But before the CAT scan, they had to find out where the blood was coming from. A day or two earlier Annette had begun to throw up blood. . So her first test was what they call a swallow. This is a test where you swallow a small amount of barium, and they take an X-ray of your throat and chest. The doctors were looking for a fistula. This is a breach between the esophagus and lung. Because Annette would start to cough whenever she drank anything, they were concerned that some of the liquid was transferring over into her lung. If this was true, it may also be the source of infection caused from bile crossing over when she threw up.

The results came with good news and bad news. The good news was a fistula did not exist. The bad news is this meant she would have to have a gastrectomy done. This is a procedure that requires you to lie on your side while the doctor shoves a tube down your throat. At the end of the tube is a camera that allows the doctor to see firsthand the condition of your stomach and esophagus. It also has a catheter that can be inserted through the tube. At the end of the catheter is a device that allows the doctor to take a sample of the tissue. This can be done either by a process that they call a brush (similar to a swab the doctor takes of your throat when they want to do a culture) or a biopsy, where they actually take a piece and send it off to pathology.

The gastrectomy showed that Annette had an ulcer on her esophagus with a viral infection in it. Antibiotics and Pepcid for the next few weeks should take care of the problem. All things considered, an ulcer is good news.

The important test we were waiting for was the CAT scan. Did the chemo work, or did Annette endure three months of being poisoned for no reason? I know I was skeptical, and I have to believe the doctors were even though they didn't say anything. Over the last three months, instead of getting better, her health was getting worse. Her energy level was diminishing, and I have been increasing her pain medication just to keep her comfortable. If it wasn't for her TPN bag she wouldn't have received any nutrition, because taking food and liquid orally was out of the question

After the CAT scan, Annette was released from the hospital. Once again, we packed up everything and went home. She was exhausted. She was always exhausted when she finally got released from the hospital. You cannot rest at a hospital; you're not there to rest. You're there to be tested and treated, and when they are done doing that, they send you home to rest. Well, this time my sweet Annette was so tired she fell asleep on the way home. When we finally made it home, I carried her from the car and right to bed. She never woke up and pretty much slept for the next two days.

I received a phone call from the doctor the morning after I brought Annette home. The news was not good. Not only did the test show that the original tumors were growing, but they had also spread, with evidence of new growth in her lungs.

I'm glad she slept for a couple days, because I spent them crying. I was without any energy. All I kept thinking was, when she wakes I'll have to tell her. Two days later Annette finally woke up. I ran a hot bath, cleaned her up, and brought her downstairs to lie on the couch. After reconnecting all of her IV lines, I brought her the medicine for her ulcer.

She asked, "What's this for?"

"Your ulcer," I replied, with a puzzled look.

"I have an ulcer?"

"Yes, that's what's causing all the nausea."

"Oh," she said.

She didn't remember. She didn't remember anything. She didn't remember throwing up blood and going to the hospital. She didn't remember the four days of tests. Nothing. She was completely void of any recollection.

Now what do I do? Do I tell her about the test results? She doesn't even remember going. It won't change anything. It's not like the cancer is going to stop or speed up. The cards are already dealt, and we don't have an ace. So I spent the next few days by her side, tending to her medication and grooming. I read to her from her daily prayer book; that always gave her comfort. We read the get-well cards as they came in and enjoyed visits from family and friends. I couldn't lie next to her, because the movement enticed the nausea, and any contact with her skin caused a cutting sensation. So I would sit on the floor next to the couch where she could see me when she opened her eyes. Sometimes she would wake up just long enough to say "hi," and sometimes I would get one of her winks.

Then, about five days later, she woke up and asked, "What did the doctor say?"

"About what?" I replied.

"The test. Did the chemo work?"

Oh, God! She remembered. I didn't know what to do. Before I could respond, of which I wasn't doing very quickly, she fell back to sleep. I didn't get much of a reprieve, though. Fifteen minutes later, she woke back up and asked again.

"What did the doctor say?"

"They didn't see what they had hoped for," I said.

"Well, at least it's not growing," she said. "Are they going to try something different?" Annette asks.

As the tears welled up in my eyes, I told her that the chemo didn't work. "It slowed the rate that it was growing, but it's still growing, and your lungs are much worse."

"When is my next treatment?" she asks.

"I don't know," I replied. "I don't think they know either. The doctor said he needs you to rest and try and build up some strength. You're too weak to receive any more chemo."

"Come and put your head on my pillow," she said.

Annette was the strength that day. She brushed my hair with her fingers as I cried into her pillow. She whispered, "I'm still here, and I'm tired, but I still want to fight."

I didn't tell her everything. I didn't have the courage to tell her that she wasn't going to win.

One week after learning that the chemo didn't work, Annette ended up back at the hospital with a fever of 103. She didn't want to go back. She was crying and pleading with me not to take her. It was extremely difficult to do, but I dressed her, and off we went just as we did many times before. If there was one thing that tore out my heart, it was seeing Annette cry. By now she accepted the fact that she was going to die from the cancer, and she didn't want to die in the hospital. I promised her that I wouldn't let that happen, but we needed to go and at least try to slow down the infection and reduce the fever.

It was Saturday night, and we spent much of the night in the emergency room. Between naps, we spent most of our time talking about nothing. At this point, she didn't have much energy and was only awake for short periods, but in the interim, it was important to both of us to keep hearing each other's voice. I would even talk to her while she was sleeping. I knew our time was growing short, and I just needed to keep letting her know that I was there. As the time grew near, it seemed we stopped talking about how much we loved each other or about the boys; these were the hard things to talk about. We seemed to focus on easier things, topics that were fun, things that might bring a smile during such a bleak time.

Dr. Kimpali came to see her Sunday afternoon. It was then that I told him that Annette had decided to stop all treatment and go home. He was saddened by the thought, but he knew it was inevitable and asked us to give them some time to at least try and get a handle on the infection so they could bring the fever down and make her comfortable. I told him that we would give them until Tuesday. He asked for Wednesday, and I agreed.

The next morning, Dr. Kimpali's partner came in during rounds with a list of strategies and a list of doctors that would be coming in to fight the fever. It was believed that Annette had another infection, but from what? Who knows? It was anyone's guess. I asked if he had talked to Dr. Kimpali yet, and he hadn't. So I informed him that Annette had decided to go home and discontinue treatment. He grabbed a chair and sat down, looked at his list, then at Annette. His face drew calm, he raised his eyebrows, and tightened his lips. I could tell by the expression on his face that he was saddened, but he understood. He had come to know Annette well, and he knew how much heart and spirit she had.

As he folded up the list and put it in his pocket, he said, "If the world only realized how great a loss this will be." It must be hard for these doctors to see the tragedy, helpless to its power. How can someone so young and vibrant, so full of hope and love and joy be ripped apart and cast aside by such a horrid disease?

After a moment, we began to make another list. This one consisted of things that needed to be done, such as making sure Annette had signed a do-not-resuscitate order, getting antibiotics to bring down the fever, and a prescription for morphine drops to fight the pain. We both looked at Annette and could see in her eyes that she was done fighting.

As promised, we were discharged from the hospital on Wednesday morning. As I prepared Annette for the ride home, ideas were racing through my mind as how to make her last days as beautiful as possible. So I thought I would start by taking the long way home, the scenic route. I wanted to share the beauty of nature with her one last time.

When we got into the car, she reached over and said, "Honey, I just want to go home."

All she wanted was the simple pleasure of lying down in her own bed. That was my last thread of hope. All along I knew Annette was dying, but I always carried a morsel of denial. This was the end. No longer could I dismiss it. The reality of death had reared its ugly head.

Suddenly, everything became a last. This would be the last time we would ride in the car together . . . the last time we would share a thought or a smile. Never again would we lie in bed on a spring morning and listen to the wind as it rustled the leaves of the tree, or watch the birds dance around the yard as they searched for nesting material. One day soon would be the last time I could look into her eyes and feel her love engulf my soul. This list is endless and too hard to write down.

Friday afternoon, when the boys came home from school, I sat them down and explained to them that Mom was going to die. After all that Annette and I have been through, this was probably the toughest thing to do. I can't imagine how they must have felt when I told them that their mom was going to die. All along they thought she would be OK. Everyone

79

else they knew that had cancer is doing OK. So their mom was going to be OK. When Annette first became ill, and we knew what her chances of surviving were, I explained to the boys individually that Mom may die. I don't think they really considered that as an option; nor did I. After a few brief questions, we wiped away the tears and went upstairs to the bedroom to spend time with her. It was nice. We shared memories and talked about the future and how she would watch over them and be there if they wanted to talk.

Just as we came to the point where there wasn't much left to say, Father Joe showed up to give Annette his blessing. After some prayer and a brief song, we began talking of the things the boys did together with Annette. One of the things that Annette always said was that she would leave pennies around to let us know that she was there and that she was alright. Just then, Nick leaned over and whispered in her ear, "Quarters." We all laughed.

Obviously, no one wanted Annette to die. Annette surely didn't want to die. But there is nothing you can do. You are helpless. You feel so small and feeble. Here lies my wife slowly dying before me, and there wasn't anything else left to do but wait. It was perfect timing with Father Joe coming when he did. By the time he had finished, we were all feeling much better about this entire situation. As strange as it may seem, this was good. Through all the turmoil and agony, in the end we had peace.

That night, all of Annette's family came over. Bill removed Annette's PICC line from her arm and gave me last instructions for administering the morphine, which was basically give her whatever she needs to eliminate the pain. I think Annette believed that once the PICC line was removed she would just die—kind of like turning off the life-support machine—because at one point, she woke up, looked around, and asked, "What are you all doing here?" as if we were in heaven with her.

That night was special for the both of us. For the first time in months we were able lie next to each other. I could hold her without causing any pain from the PICC line or from the tumor in her back or ribs, thanks to the morphine. Saturday morning, she woke me to take her to the bathroom. When we returned to the bed, she lay next to me with her head on my chest. It was wonderful and peaceful. I talked to her for nearly two hours. She would doze off from time to time, but I just kept talking. It was so wonderful being able to hold her again. Do you know that feeling of peaceful joy when a baby sleeps soundly as it lies on your chest? That's how it was that morning. I felt as though Annette was like a baby, putting absolute trust in me to care for her while she rested. The love I felt for her that morning was a thousand times greater than I have ever felt before. As strange as it may seem, I knew as she slept that she was collecting all the love I could give her, as if she was gathering it in her soul to carry with her when she moved into the next world.

After a while she woke and said in a soft, peaceful voice, "Why don't you take a shower and get cleaned up?"

"Are you sure?" I ask.

She nodded her head and said, "Go on. It's alright."

"OK," I said. "Just a quick one, though, and I'll be right back."

"Take your time," she replied. "I'll be alright."

"Why don't I call your mom up? I know she's waiting to see you."

Annette smiled and said, "Yeah, that would be nice."

So I called her mother up to be with her while I took a quick shower. I came out of the bathroom talking, just as if we were getting up on a Sunday preparing for the day. Then I noticed it was strangely quiet. I turned and looked. Annette's mom was standing at the end of the bed. Her expression was empty as she held her hand over her mouth. I squeezed her hand as I passed by her. Annette's breathing was very shallow, and her eyes were rolled back in her head. I sat next to her on the bed and held her hand as she took her last breath. Thinking back on it, I wonder why I didn't lie beside her and hold her or sit next to her and place her head on my chest for those last few moments. I guess I didn't because this wasn't Hollywood, and I didn't have time to think what may be the most touching way to spend the last moments together. Essentially, I was in shock, and all I could do was sit next to her and hold her hand. This is life, not a movie, and life isn't always grandiose and heart-touching. At times, it is cold and cruel, while other times are warm and compassionate.

I realize now that when Annette woke and asked me to go and take a shower, she knew it was her time to go. I have learned that this happens a lot. A person such as myself will spend months next to the one they love, providing every need and cherishing every second. Then, in the few moments that you are out of the room, the person you love so deeply passes away. It is almost as if they know it's time, and they understand that the separation would be less painful if we weren't there to witness the moment that they pass into this unconscious state. My love for Annette goes beyond the boundaries of our universe. So even though I only held her hand, I'm sure my love for her enveloped her tired body, and she felt the security of my love as she passed on to the other side.

On Saturday, March 29, 2003, at 10:30 a.m., Annette Ciaramella left this world peacefully in her own bed with me and her mother by her side.

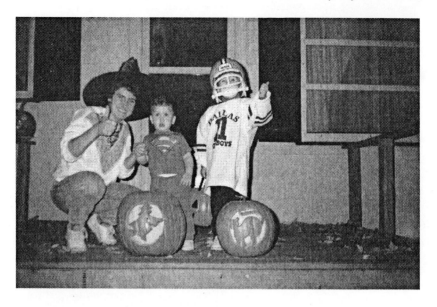

Halloween 1993

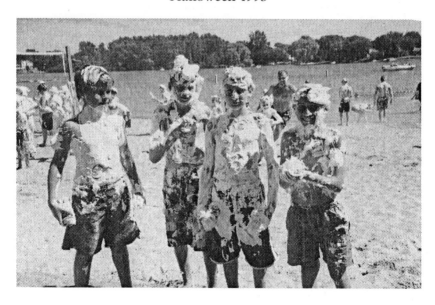

Nick, Zack, and Jake, victorious in the annual shaving cream fight

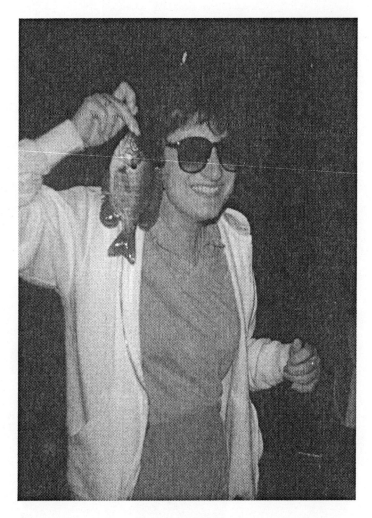

Annette's the only keeper in this picture

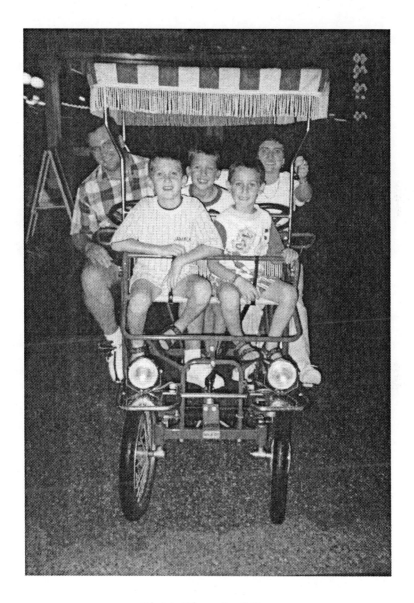

Living life to the fullest

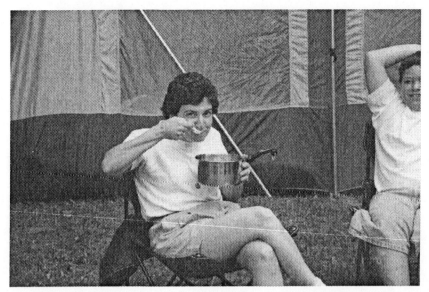

Dining Out

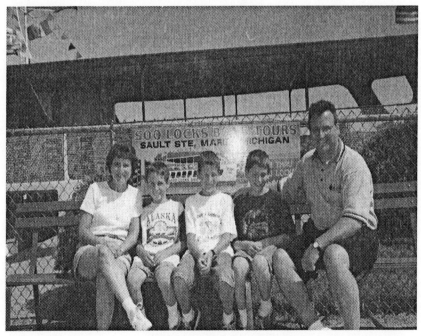

At the Soo Locks in Michigan

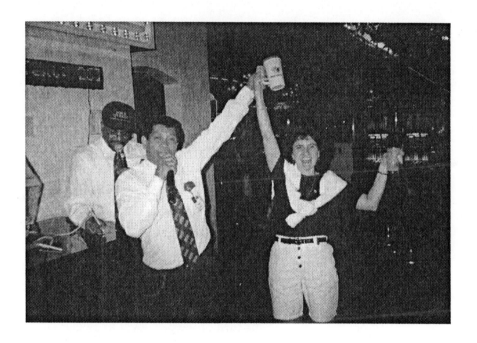

Winning big in Las Vegas

Chapter 2

My Wife, Our Life

Annette was born April 23, 1962. Like me, she was the middle child of five. She has three sisters and one brother. Joann is the eldest, then Angela with Sam and Lisa round out the pack. Annette was the feisty one—very sharp and witty. There wasn't much that you were going to get past her. She was street-smart and shrewd. Annette carried the title of "spitfire." I'm not sure who tagged her with that name, but it certainly fit. She stood 4 feet 11½ inches tall. She always claimed five feet, but I would never give her the half inch. When I was around, I always made sure the record was right. That was our little thing. Every couple has their little teases, and this was mine. These days, I give her the half inch; it just doesn't matter anymore. As I mentioned before, she weighed in at 105 pounds, and every bit of it is toned up and in shape.

Annette's childhood was spent growing up in a small suburb of Detroit called Harper Woods. It's a nice little town with clean streets lined with ranch-style brick homes. Like most young girls, Annette was involved in dance class, Brownies, and other after-school activities. Her maiden name is Castiglione, which stands for Castle of the Lion—at least, that's what her dad always claimed. Her great grandparents on her mother's side made the journey from Sicily around the turn of the century. I knew her Great Grandmother Antoinette as Mama Donnia and her Great Grandfather Jesepi, who died before I met Annette, was called Papa Beppi. Annette came from a large Italian family, and they're all named after the parents and grandparents. On Annette's mother's side, the boys (and I'm talking about multiple generations) are named Peter, Paul, or Joseph, and the girls are Annette and Antoinette. Conversations were always confusing, mostly because you spend half of it figuring out who the heck you're talking about. For example, you have Uncle Peter's Peter's Peter.

Despite this obsession of naming their children after one another, this is the kindest, most generous group of people you will ever meet. They are active in their church and community, and there's always room for another plate at the dinner table. The funny thing about the Italian people is that they are either very kind and generous or so tight that they make Jack Benny look like Santa Claus. There isn't a middle ground; it is either one way or the other.

Thankfully, Annette's family is of the generous nature. They are a lot of fun to be around and will support you whenever they can. Annette's dad worked his way up through Chrysler from the trash department to interior designer. He took classes at night, worked in a few job shops to get design experience, and secured a position in Chrysler's interior-design department. John was what you would call a go-to man. He had a knack for making contacts and building relationships with people in other departments. When it came time to get a certain material or report in order to get a job done, the other members of the department would come to him to come up with the goods. When he retired, his fellow workers presented him with the John Castiglione Award. It was a set of plans rolled up with a grip made of clay wrapped around the center—ergonomically correct, I might add. You see, if you're off scrounging up a report or some type of material for your department, you're less likely to be stopped or questioned if you're carrying something like a set of plans or a box or bag, something that made you look like you were actually supposed to be where you were at. Well, his favorite prop was a set of plans, and he never went anywhere without them. He took pride in helping whomever he could. Many a student or coworker owed thanks to him for his help on a project or getting them what they needed to get them out of whatever situation they were in. To give you an example, I had a friend in the air force who was an engineer, and when he was getting ready to be discharged, my father-in-law spent three weeks lining up interviews, one of which turned into a job. All this for someone he never met.

Annette's mother was the quintessential housewife. It was her job to keep the house running smoothly, and she did. Amazingly enough, she managed to keep the house well supplied with food and essentials with the meager allowance that was given to her. I'm sure this is where Annette learned her skill of stretching a dollar. There was never anything out of place; the home was spotless and organized. She ironed the bedsheets, for crying out loud! And she can cook. And cook, and cook. As soon as the breakfast dishes were cleaned up, she would start on lunch or dinner, depending on what day it was. Annette's mom is a wonderful person. She is always willing to help and lend a hand. She has many friends and family that know they can count on her for just about anything.

I remember the first holiday dinner I attended. You would think that the other brothers-in-laws would have clued me in, but I think they enjoyed the surprise just as much as her family did. You see, on a holiday, food is presented all day. This is the only family I know that takes pictures of the holiday turkey and frames it on the wall. I'm not kidding. Do you know those picture frames that have about ten different areas of different shapes and sizes? Well, when you walk into the family room from the garage, there, hanging on the wall in one of the areas, is a picture of a holiday turkey.

Anyway, after gorging ourselves on shrimp and other appetizers, we are called to the table for dinner. First we have soup followed by a pasta dish. Not realizing what is to come, I have a pretty good-sized portion of both. Next comes the main dish. This particular time they were having lemon chicken with potatoes, two vegetables, and bread. Oh, I forgot to mention the dinner salad. Seeing that this is the first time at Annette's house for a holiday dinner, I wasn't going to insult her mother and grandmother— her Italian mother and grandmother—by not taking full helpings. Now, her mom wouldn't say anything, but Grandma wouldn't hesitate to say, "Watsa matta, you no like?" Meaning, if you don't have three helpings, you must not like the food she spent eight hours preparing.

After an hour of food flying and dishes clanging, I thought I had survived. My stomach was ready to burst. I rolled off the chair and made it to the couch, knowing that the slightest movement would cause my belly to burst like an overfilled water balloon.

It wasn't but ten minutes later when Sam came over and said, "It's time to play Tripoley and eat dessert."

I lifted my head and looked at him through half-closed eyes and said, "You have got to be kidding."

He said, "No, we play every time we get together."

"No," I said. "What do you mean 'dessert'?"

"Oh, yeah. Ma and Grandma made three special desserts just because you're here. We don't always get Blanc Mange (Pronounced Bionge Mugadi) (a white cream gelled dessert with nuts and cherries)."

"OK . . . OK, I'm coming."

Once again, one serving wouldn't do. Three servings later they finally cleared away the dessert dishes and brought out the ham and bread for sandwiches. That's right, ham sandwiches. My eyes rolled back as I fell over onto Annette's lap. I could hear them chuckling and giggling.

Then Chuck (Joann's husband) said, "I never made it to dessert."

Well, I'll tell you what. When Annette's younger sister Lisa brought Jeff Williams, who is now Lisa's husband, over for his first holiday dinner, I didn't say a word!

Most of the stories that are told around the kitchen table that have been recalled time and time again all seem to have been about their vacations at their cabin located on Wildwood Lake in northern Michigan. Wildwood Lake was originally a stream that passed through a small valley. At some point in time, trees were cleared from the valley and surrounding hills, and a dam was built at the south end of the stream, creating a large inland lake that is great for water-skiing, fishing, or a quiet leisurely cruise at dusk. There is a peninsula that comes up through the center of the lake from the south, dividing it into two halves. Lush grassy knolls and hills are lined with large pine, maple, and oak trees that surround the lake. It is a tranquil place, even though all the lots were sold, and a small golf course was built on the outlying area. The way the lots are laid out between hills and ridges makes it quiet and very relaxing.

As I mentioned before, Annette was the daredevil of the family, the spitfire. She never hesitated to take on a challenge. I remember the story where she and her siblings decided to go horseback riding. Annette was ten years old when she volunteered to ride "Red." Red was what you would call a temperamental beast. At forty years old, Annette weighed 105 pounds; imagine what she weighed at the age of ten. Anyway, this particular trip ended up with Red deciding that he had had enough, and it was time to head for the barn—at a full gallop, I might add. At this point on the trail, the barn was about a mile away, around the bend and over the hill. I have been in this situation myself, and there isn't a thing you can do except hang on for dear life. That horse is not going to stop until it is ready to, and they usually don't come to a gradual stop—they stop very abruptly. The following week, she was back at it again. Annette always claimed she got back on Red to prove to herself that she could do it. I think she wanted to show Red that she wasn't afraid of him. That's how she was; ask anyone who knew Annette. She didn't care how big and bad you were. If she felt you needed it, she brought you down a couple of notches.

Not to get off the subject, but there was an incident when we lived in Las Vegas where she was rear-ended by another car on the way home from work. They both got out and looked, and on the outside, there didn't appear to be any damage. Not thinking, she left without getting any information from the driver. When she came home and told me what happened, we did a more thorough investigation and found the trunk was buckled along with other damage. Well, for the next two weeks she timed her travel home so as to possibly come across the guy that hit her. I have to tell you, I knew nothing of this. Amazingly enough, she ran across the man that hit her, and she followed him home to confront him and get his information for the insurance. Naturally, he told her to get lost. Well, she wrote down his address and sent it to the insurance company. The thing is, this guy lived in the seediest side of town. I think a lineman in the NFL would have had second thoughts about going into this neighborhood, but not Annette. About a month later, we get a letter from the insurance company stating that their notices were being returned with "No such person living at this address." Annette wants to go back and confront the guy! It took three hours to convince her that it wasn't worth it. All she could see was that this guy wasn't being responsible, and that enraged her to the bone.

Back to "up north." You have to live in Michigan to understand that phrase. It doesn't matter where you vacation in the state. If you travel more than one mile north of where your home is, you are going "up north." What can I say? We're a weird lot here. But what the heck! We have the majority of the fresh-water supply for the entire United States within our borders.

Another story she liked to tell was about the time when she was water-skiing with the neighbors one hot summer day. It became even hotter when she came out of the water with her bathing-suit top around her waist. She thought all the boys on the boat were cheering because she got up on the skis so easily. She soon realized she was exhibiting much more than just her athletic ability, and let go of the rope. Taking things in stride, she fixed her top, waited for the boat to come around, and grabbed onto the rope for another go. Truth be known, she probably enjoyed the attention—at least a little bit.

Every time we went fishing out on that lake she would tell me about the time she took her cousins fishing. There was Peter, Paul, Joe, Peter, Annette, and her other two cousins, both named Annette. The reason she tells me this is because she likes me to bait her hooks now, claiming she did a lifetime of hook baiting when she took her cousins fishing, and it was her turn to be pampered. This is Annette's idea of being pampered, having someone else bait her fishhook. What a woman!

The remark that seems to be relayed to me quite often these past few months is "I didn't realize how close you and Annette were" or "I didn't realize how much of a team you two were." These are words from other couples. I guess I'm just as ignorant to the fact that many other couples didn't share the same kind of relationship that we did.

I didn't realize how blessed I was to have a relationship with a woman that was as much a part of me as I was a part of her. We shared everything. You may ask, What do you mean everything? And I tell you, everything. I don't even know how to begin. Not only did we support each other when making crucial decisions, we also worked together to make every day special. We never said good-bye; it was always "I'll see you later." I stole that from my parents, my Dad never told my Mom goodbye, it was always "see you later", We planned everything. When I say we planned everything, I don't mean that we planned our day down to the minute and followed a strict schedule. When I say planned . . . well, here's an example. The boys love spareribs—baby backs, to be specific. However, they're quite expensive. Every once in a while, Annette would call me at work to tell me she had picked some up because they were on sale. That's great, but we wouldn't stop there. She would say, "How about having them on Friday night?" I would agree and then add, "Let's get a movie." Then she may say, "I could pick up a few more, and each of the boys could invite a friend. We'll make a party out of it." We always tried to put a little twist into those special occasions. Most of the time, we didn't plan anything major. Just a touch to make it fun.

We would start planning our next vacation on the plane home from the one we were just on. Some people thought we were nuts, never satisfied. But we were; we were very satisfied. We thrived on the anticipation of the trip or the fun meal or going to the movies or having company over. After a while, things begin to overlap, and the next thing you know, you have developed this relationship where everyday life becomes one big event.

I have been told by some that their marriage has stifled. Everyday life is boring. I don't understand that. They are living in the same home with their best friend in the entire world, and they find that boring. You can say whatever you feel, you can do whatever you want together, you can love and touch and be together without any inhibitions, and you're bored? Oh, how blessed we were. This is what hurts the most. I had the ideal world with Annette as my wife, and I lost her. We lost each other. I hope on the other side she can only feel the love and not the sorrow. I talk to her constantly, hoping that if she can hear me she will know that I am going to be alright, and some day we will be together again. I still can't imagine doing all the things we did together without her. Because we did everything together.

In My Opinion

These next several paragraphs address adult relationships and are very opinionated. I wasn't sure about putting this section in, but after talking to a few friends, they thought I should. I don't claim to be an expert on relationships, and the only firsthand knowledge I have is my marriage to Annette. Annette and I have had friends come to us over the years when they were having problems. Sometimes they came for advice, and sometimes they came just to talk. They came because they knew whatever they said would be kept in the strictest confidence. The relationship that Annette and I shared was unique, very special, and blessed. Our marriage wasn't good— it was great. It was magnificent. That is not an opinion; that is a fact, a fact supported by everyone who knew us. I still don't know what I did prior to meeting Annette that afforded me the gift to love and be loved by such a generous and giving angel.

I'm asked, "What made your relationship with Annette so special?"
I would reply, "The way we made love."
That usually gets a very strange look. Annette and I made love every minute we were together. Every time we smiled at each other or caressed the other's face. A kiss on the neck or a hug from behind. A phone call to say "I'm on my way home," or a special surprise. Telling the other "my love for you is eternal, and regardless of what happens, you are and will be the light of my soul for ever and ever." If you think you don't hear it from your spouse, all you have to do is listen a little closer. The love is there; it was there in the beginning and is still there today. The problem is you let the rest of your life interfere with the one reason you came together in the first place. Our relationship grew the way it did, because we always focused on what we could do for the other as opposed to what the other was doing for me. We were always cultivating our marriage, never harvesting.

The word "soulmate" has become the catchphrase of recent past. It always amazed us when we would hear someone say "he is my soulmate" or "she is my soulmate," only to hear them follow up with a "BUT . . ." For example, "She is my soulmate, but she drives me nuts when she does—" . . . what ever she does. If you truly have a soulmate there are no

95

"buts." It's as simple as that. Not to say that you will never disagree on a certain subject or that you never have an argument or a fight. Soulmates do encounter these things; they have to, or they aren't being honest to each other. And if you have truly found your soulmate, then his or her little quirks don't bother you, and they certainly don't rate a "but."

While I'm on the subject of relationships, it grinds me when people say that in a good relationship you should never go to bed angry. That's a crock. There's nothing wrong with being mad for a while. It doesn't mean you don't love each other. All it means is you don't agree on something. To build a fence and say you can't sleep until you resolve this only creates stress and resentment. That's right, resentment. Correct me if I'm wrong, but what ends up happening is someone has to give in and admit he or she was wrong, whether they feel they were or not. And that builds resentment. Sleep on the issue. Give yourself room to step back and review the other's opinion. There are times that you may agree to just disagree. That builds respect, not resentment.

After Annette's funeral, many people came to me and said, "We never realized how close you were" or "The two of you have taught us the importance of remembering to keep the sparks going that drew us together in the first place." What was our secret? you may ask. It was love, plain and simple. We made love every chance we had. Not just physical sex, although I'll get to that in a minute. I'm talking about being aware of your spouse twenty-four hours a day. Pick up the phone (this only has to be **_once_**) during the day and let her/him know that you love them. Buy a single rose from time to time. Brush your hand across their back or bottom (which was always my favorite landing zone). Send a wink and a smile from across the room. Help fold the clothes or get the kids off to bed. Let the dinner dishes go for an hour and go for a walk (hand in hand). The bottom line is, cherish the time you have. Your relationship is the most important factor of your marriage. Think about it. Love is the reason you married in the first place; desire will keep it alive and strong.

Physical sex is what fuels the desire and creates the bond of trust, which over time is impenetrable. Stay with me here. Many couples allow work and kids and all of their extracurricular activities to interfere with their sex life. DON'T LET IT! Physical sex is the most satisfying, stress-relieving, relationship-bonding activity that a couple can do together—and it's **FREE**.

The act itself allows you to bare your souls to each other. There are probably many of us here that, when in the midst of sex, feel alive and vigorous as we did when we were twenty. We all get in a conversation from time to time where someone says, "Can you picture Mom and Dad doing the nasty?" And everyone goes, "EWWW!" And someone blurts out, "Too much info," as they wave their hands frantically or cover their ears. But guess what? Our kids are saying the same about us. And our parents said the same about theirs. So you see, it doesn't matter how old and wrinkled you are when it comes to sex; in our minds, we all see ourselves as young and vibrant.

The preparation for sex in itself opens the door for communication, and communication is the foundation of a healthy relationship. Think about it. The first thing you do is you peel away all material things. You come together with love and desire, separated only by the suit you were given at birth. You accept each other's imperfections openly.

With all of today's material possessions cast aside, you join together in a union of love that allows you to be who you really are. During the act of love all inhibition and fears are put aside. Words are said or whispered in your mate's ear that you would never dream of saying in public. Your bodies create sounds as your love creates and excretes fluids. Moans, chest farts, and chirps of ecstasy riddle the room. All these things come into play whenever you make love to your partner.

The most important thing that develops, though, is humility. You see each other and yourself for who you really are. What can possibly be too embarrassing or humiliating to talk about with the person that you love, the person you vowed to cherish, the person you just spent the last thirty , fifteen, or two minutes doing the most basic, natural, first-rung–on-the-ladder-of–Species survival, primal act with? Sex with your spouse is the key that unlocks the door to communication. With communication comes a more open relationship. The more sex you share, the more lovemaking you perform and the more comfortable you will become with each other. And here is the kicker. The more comfortable you become with each other, the more comfortable you are talking to your spouse about everything and anything. That's communication. That's what leads to a closer, more desirable relationship. Which, by the way, leads to desire, and what do you want when you have desire? MORE SEX. More lovemaking, which leads to more communication. And the world turns. Before you know it, you're one of the lucky ones that has a mate that you can giggle with.

This is the one area where you can be selfish and say to your lover/ partner/mate, "I desire you, and I want you as often as I can." I just don't see how you can be turned down. We all want to be loved. We all want someone in our lives that thinks we are the one, and we are the reason they get up in the morning. And in return for this love and devotion, all I have to do is make love to the person that I love and desire more than anyone else on this entire planet. If you think this sounds good but question, Who has the time to have sex three, four, five, or even six to seven times a week? Well, let me tell you from personal experience. You do. We all do. All you have to do is allow yourself the freedom to desire. Be assertive. Act on your desire. Take the initiative. Love is the passion of the world. Grab as much of it as you can, and you will become one of the wealthiest couples of your generation. Annette and I found the secret to building our relationship was a thing that is referred to as a quickie. A quickie gives just as much satisfaction as an hour-long session (fifty-five minutes of foreplay included, of course). And like a small snack between meals, it's not meant to be the staple of the relationship, but it's a means of keeping the flame burning until it's time to come to the table.

Romance is an important factor. Everyone likes to be romanced; it makes you feel special. So don't forget to romance each other throughout the day. Yeah, that's right: throughout the day. Marriage is an 86,400-second-a-day commitment—a wonderful commitment at that. It's the greatest endeavor that you can embark on. It was the romance that fed the fires of passion. We were open and free with each other. We came together because we wanted to be there. It is important to be open and loving. Let your mate know that you want to be there. Let him or her know that you're not there just because it's the second Tuesday of the month. Always keep in mind that this is not a one-sided expedition. Show your lover that you care by asking what position they prefer. Get to know what stimulates your mate. Find out what they desire in order to reach the finish line. And most of all, be truthful to one another, and be open to make or consider suggestions that will make it better. Let loose of your inhibitions. Let your spouse/lover know what your fantasies are. Don't be afraid to say or ask for what you want or need, regardless of how out of character you may think it to be. There are plenty of people out there that, when in public, are quiet and shy, proper and respectable. But when it comes to sex, they are wild and imaginative. Tell your partner exactly what your fantasy is. You may be surprised at the response. You may very well find that when making love you both are out of character. Who knows, you both may have the same kind of fantasy, or your fantasies may complement your partner's.

Mix it up. There is a reason why a band or D J will play both fast and slow songs. If you don't mix it up, boredom will set in. The bedroom door is closed. Be free to have fun. For that matter, be free to have fun in any room you desire. In my opinion, there is nothing more exciting than imaginative sex. It's like walking into your favorite restaurant. You know what's on the main menu, but you never know what the special is until you get there.

Sex should be fun, plain and simple. It is the greatest gift we were given to share with each other. Work on both your physical and emotional relationship as hard if not harder than you would on your career, and it will reap rewards that far exceed your expectations.

Once again, I'm not claiming to be an expert. All I know is that Annette and I had a beautiful marriage, and our physical relationship not only opened the door to uninhibited communication, but it was the cement that bonded our love. Regardless of the day we were having, at the end, we would come together, putting aside everyone and everything to be with each other—her and I alone, just the two of us. It was these times that reinforced the bond that made us one.

Like I said, the question was asked, so I answered it. One last thought before I go on. Not that I would ever wish what has happened to Annette and me on anyone else. But if couples could experience just for a brief moment the loss, they would realize how blessed they are to have found a best friend and mate to share an entire lifetime of love. To have children and watch them grow into adults and start families of their own. To have a confidant to share their most intimate thoughts and desires. To know your spouse is there to laugh and cry with. To be there when you need a safe haven or a foundation that will support you. Oh, how I miss my angel.

Gifts

Annette and I have an unusual relationship when it comes to gift giving and the expression of our love. She doesn't like cut flowers; she feels they are a waste of money. So we plant flowers all round the house during the summer and open the windows to let the fragrance in. To the disbelief of most of our friends, we don't exchange gifts on Christmas, anniversaries, birthdays, Valentine's Day, Sweetest Day, or any other day that society has deemed essential for the giving of a gift in order to express your love and honor. We never understood what giving a gift had to do with showing your love and admiration for each other. We would exchange cards—sometimes they were bought, sometimes they were handmade, and other times it was a quick note jotted down on a scrap piece of paper. For example, on our anniversary I might stop and pick up a card and her favorite candy bar for a mere $3.50. Now I could have shown my love by spending $100 on a gift, but it wouldn't express my love to her any better. Think about it: what does it take to go out and buy a card and a dozen roses or clothing or even jewelry? It doesn't take any more time to buy or even give. It truly is the thought that counts. Instead of using money to express my love, I can give time—my time—out of my day. As we are very aware of now, even more than we were before Annette was stricken with cancer, time spent together on this earth is much more valuable than any amount of money. So if I want to really express myself, I could give her a half-hour massage that night after I clean up the dinner dishes and get the kids off to bed. These are the kind of things that strengthened our relationship. You see, we don't wait for a date on the calendar to dictate when we should show our devotion to each other. Christmas, birthdays, anniversaries, and all of the other commercially generated holidays are mere dates on a calendar. We don't need a calendar, nor do we wait for a date on one to celebrate our marriage. We celebrate every day of the year.

I'm not saying we never buy each other gifts. It's just that we learned that giving gifts on dictated dates has absolutely no bearing on our relationship. It isn't important that we go out on our anniversary for a romantic evening. We may do something two weeks later when it is more convenient, when we can relax and enjoy the night. Or we may do nothing at all, depending on what is going on at the time between work, the kids, or school. Besides, we found that we grew closer by taking a weekend away.

Once or twice a year, we would go to Las Vegas or somewhere we could get away from everyone. This included the kids, family, and work. It was time that we could spend focusing on our relationship. The time spent was more important than any gift that could be bought. The memory of the long weekend will last much longer than a dozen roses.

People say they can't afford to go out of town two times a year. Well, if you add up the money you spend on gifts over a year, there is plenty of money. Keep in mind, you don't have to fly or even go far. We have shared wonderful weekends within fifty miles of our home. In fact, we have spent weekends at home. Talk to your family and friends, and see if any of them would be interested in trading times watching each other's children. You will find good friends that you can trust to watch your children, and you can have a glorious time at very little expense. It is the time, not the cost or the place. We even enjoy surprising our friends with this idea. From time to time, we will call a friend and tell them that we are picking their kids up for the weekend, and they should start planning a getaway. Sometimes it takes a bit of persuasion, but we have never been turned down. We also hope that we are teaching our boys that the value of a relationship isn't based on material things, but based on feelings and dedication to each other and the trust you build between you.

As with most relationships, over time we learned what really is appreciated, and throughout the year, you will come across those things that you can do for each other. For example, Annette likes a special kind of chili on her hot dogs. When she was young, her family would go for a drive downtown to a diner called Lafayette Coney Island. This is quite the place; there is nothing fancy at all about it. You sit either at the counter or at long white tables lined up one after the other. The server asks you for your order. There are no menus; the list is very basic. As you give him your order, he yells it to the guy behind the counter. If you ever saw the "Pepsi/Chips" skit on Saturday Night Live, you would have thought that this was where they got the idea. Maybe they did. If I'm not mistaken, some of the cast spent time working at Second City. So whenever the opportunity presented itself, I would get some chili to go, stop and get some hot dogs with the skins, and surprise her with a meal that she only gets once or twice a year.

Now I could drive down and get the chili whenever I wanted, but that would take the fun out of it. It would no longer be special. That chili dog meant more to her than a dinner in a five-star restaurant. It's not that she doesn't like being pampered at an expensive restaurant, but she knows that in the middle of my day I thought of her and put her above whatever I was doing to get the chili and dogs. We enjoy going to the movies, but with the cost of babysitting, it makes going to the movies impractical. We will spend $12 on the movie and $40 on babysitting and another $20 in extras. So we save that time for when we go on our weekend getaway. It is something we share together and look forward to. So, you see, we don't get each other these little gifts because some date on the calendar dictates it. We do it because we had the opportunity to go a little out of the way and show the other that we were thinking about them. And when you have that thought guiding your actions, it doesn't have to be grandiose. The simplest idea creates mountains of strength, trust, and love that solidifies your relationship together.

Annette was a stay-at-home mom. By the way, don't ever tell a stay-at-home mom that she doesn't have a job. Just because she doesn't get dressed and go work in an office somewhere doesn't mean that she doesn't have a job. Stay-at-home moms and dads have the toughest job out there, and I'm glad Annette stepped up to the challenge.

People say we are rich because we can afford to live off of one income and still do all the things we do. We aren't rich, and I don't make a wealth of money. I make a moderate income. The reason we don't have money problems is because of Annette's ability to manage money. She has a knack for finding deals and creating them when they aren't necessarily there. Sometimes it gets a little embarrassing, so I will generally just step aside and let her do her thing. I remember when we bought our boat. We had settled on a price with the salesman at the dealer, but the day we were supposed to pick it up he called and said he wouldn't be able to come through with one of his promises. Well, she made him pay dearly for it.

Knowing he had to move the boat before the end of the year and casting doubt on his integrity, she had convinced him to take another $1,000 off the price. I used to let these things bother me, but if he really couldn't afford to take the extra money off, he wouldn't have. Besides, we are very loyal customers. The dealer is an hour away from us, and there are probably twenty-five dealers between our house and his dealership, but we go there for everything from tune-ups to polish, and we refer them to everyone we can. So, you see, he may have given up a little in the beginning, but he has made it back tenfold. She can also stretch a dollar like you wouldn't believe.

There are times when she comes home from shopping, and the stores have actually paid her for taking the item home with her. For example, she bought a CD player for one of the boys. She had a coupon from the Entertainment Book for so much off any item over $25, waited for it to go on sale, and also had a manufacturer's rebate coupon. By the time she was done, she had the CD player and $3.59 to boot.

One day I came home from work and was treated to the modeling of a very sexy evening outfit that Annette had bought for the Disney Cruise that we had planned. Always at the end of these demonstrations I would have to guess what she had paid. It's kind of like a miniature version of The Price is Right If I guess right, I win a prize that I won't get into telling you about. Anyway, this particular outfit sold for $125, and she paid $3. That's right, $3. I don't know how she does it, but you can ask anyone she knows, and they will tell you that she is always dressed tastefully and in style—and she does it for pennies on the dollar.

It's not just her clothes—all of us are clothed for just pennies. She can smell a bargain or sale miles away. One of her secrets is to shop the garage sales in the more affluent neighborhoods. Many times she will come home with clothes for me or the boys that still have the tags on them; they have never been worn. Yet she pays $2 for a $40 shirt or pair of pants.

I do have a story for you, and I think you'll get a kick out of it.

We were planning a trip to visit our friends in Chicago. We have been there many times before, but this trip was a little different. For the first time, we had made plans to leave the kids at home, and the four of us would go out to dinner. Well, on this trip we were going to a seafood joint. Not a real fancy place, but dinner for four would run $125 to $150. For whatever the reason, Annette just couldn't decide what pair of shoes she was going to take for this dinner out. For four days she kept flip-flopping, right up to the day we left when I finally said, "Pick a pair. I'm closing the suitcase."

The big night came. It was raining, so John dropped the girls off at the door, and he and I went and parked the car. We had an early reservation, and the girls were seated immediately. As John and I made our way to the table, we could see them laughing. Not only were they laughing uncontrollably, but they were looking directly at us. Any guy will tell you that under these circumstances, the very first thing he would do is check his zipper. We did, and the barn door was securely latched. We wondered now what could be so funny. When we reached the table, John asks without delay, "What's so funny, Tam?" By this time, we're laughing, and we didn't even know why.

Tammy says, "You have to look under the table."

"Why?" we asked.

"Just look," she said.

So we leaned over, lifted the tablecloth, and looked around. Sitting back up, John and I looked at each other, and then back at Tammy.

"So what's so funny?"

Now, both Tammy and Annette are just roaring.

"Look again," Tammy says. "Look at Annette's feet."

Before we could look again, Tammy blurts out as if we are on the other side of the room, "Annette has her slippers on!"

That's right, after four days of turmoil over these dumb shoes, she walked out of the house with her slippers on. We laughed about it all night.

As you all know, it is customary when someone passes on that small gifts or personal possessions of the deceased are given to family and close friends as remembrances. After Annette died, I couldn't come up with a gift for John and Tammy. Then one day, when I was going through Annette's things, I came across those slippers, and I knew on the spot what to do with them. So I packaged them up with a few other items that I needed to mail and sent them off to Chicago for safekeeping.

My wife was a big Oprah fan, and I remember one time Oprah had this lady on her show that fed her family for $2 a day, or something like that—but, heck, she was feeding them red beans and rice for dinner! Annette was feeding the five of us for close to that, and we were eating steak. She goes to the grocery store, and between sales and coupons, it is rare that she doesn't save at least 40 percent off her bill. We don't have money problems, not because I make a lot of money, but because she takes her job very seriously. Like everything Annette did, her heart and soul goes into it. Whether it's buying clothes and food for the family or building our relationship, I could never claim she wasn't giving it her all.

She always said, get involved in the community, become part of your kids' life. Annette and I always volunteered to help out at school, church, or our homeowners association. If a teacher needed someone to help out in class or chaperone a field trip, Annette was there. The kids had a program where they collect soup labels and earn points to buy things for the school. Annette and a few of her friends organized and counted up the labels for the entire school. By counting the labels and organizing them, not only did the school meet the criteria from the manufacturers, but they also determine which class donated the most labels every month, and, in turn, that class received a prize of some sort. This is just one of the many things that she got involved in at school.

Annette made life beautiful. She was so full of energy and wit. Whenever we had plans to do something or go somewhere, she would have the day planned out with little ditties along the way to make it interesting. She always knew when and where something was happening. If she wasn't taking the boys to Chuck E. Cheese's with their report cards for free tokens, she was signing us all up for a free dessert on our birthday at the local restaurants. Even when she was planning our wedding reception, somehow she found out about this hall that just changed ownership. She went and sampled the food and locked in a price that was $8 a plate less than all of the other halls in the surrounding area, and the food was great. Every so often she would pick up someone's favorite dessert or get a movie that we were looking forward to seeing but never seemed to get around to watching. If she found chicken or steak on sale, she would buy enough for two families and make dinner for the neighbors. Annette was always thinking ahead about what she could do that would bring a little cheer into your life. I don't think we (and when I say "we" I mean the community as a whole) realize how much we are going to miss all that she did.

Annette was loved and still is loved, by many people. She had touched so many lives and brought so much joy to so many. Many of the kids in the neighborhood knew her because of her work at church and with the beach staff in our neighborhood. She loved going down to the beach. In our association, anyone under age thirteen has to be accompanied by an adult, so when she went down to the beach, she would take any kids we knew with her, provided they behaved—and they did, because they knew they wouldn't go the next time if they didn't.

We have a wonderful association in our neighborhood. They have many activities throughout the year for the families and the kids. Like any organization, they rely heavily on volunteers to get the work done. Whether it is beach cleanup in the spring or working a booth on Kids' Day, she was always there. In addition to volunteering at the beach, she is the assistant treasurer for our homeowners association, a den mother, a member of the activities committee at our church, and a room mom at the boys elementary school.

There is a "moms" group at our church that Annette belongs to. Once a week, they get together and discuss a chapter out of their book. For the most part, they discuss relationships and how they are linked to church and God. Because of her involvement in the community, Annette and I have a wealth of support. During Annette's illness, there was so much help I didn't know what to do with them. Now that things are settling down, I look back, and I don't know what I would have done without them.

Chapter 3

Support

Dear Everyone,

Before I get started here, I want to say thank you to all family members, friends, coworkers, church members, and the rest of the community that came together and rallied behind our family as we traveled down this relentless road of ambiguity and hopelessness. I could live to be a thousand years old, and it wouldn't be enough time to repay the kindness, understanding and generosity that all of you showered us with. What you did, you did out of love and compassion. You demonstrated the essential good that is in all people and confirmed our belief that when things get tough you can depend on the support of those around you. Community is the heart of civilized society. All of you are not the norm; you have set the standard for others to follow. We are blessed to have received such a gracious gift.

May the angels in heaven above enter your lives, and let their radiance bring the joy and protection of God's love to you and your families.

Love
The Ciaramella
Family

I have never been the type of person to ask for help, so when Annette became ill it took awhile before I was able to accept help from anyone. All along there were friends and family that would step in and take care of the boys. That was a must. I had to have someone there for them, or I would have been a neglectful parent. What I'm talking about is having people come in and clean the house, go shopping, run the boys to hockey, bring dinner over, or just stop by so I could have a break and take a nap.

We went through different stages of this. In the beginning, I refused all help. Partially because I didn't know what I needed done, but most of all, it was that I didn't want to impose on anybody. I didn't want to be in anyone's debt. Always willing to provide help, but never willing to accept it.

With three boys in the house, it didn't take long before the cupboards began to empty and the laundry started piling up. It's not that I wasn't addressing it; it was just building up quicker than I could take care of it. So I opened the doors and began to accept help from family and friends. It was like opening the floodgates. The phone constantly rang with everyone wanting to know what to do. Then there were the ones that just took it upon themselves to decide what we needed. Bags of groceries would be left on the porch. Dinners would show up unexpectedly. I came home, and there were six women in the house cleaning things and putting stuff away. It was running rampant, out of control. Dinners were showing up ten minutes after we just ate. I had so much food coming in, there was no place left to put it. A lot of people sent baked goods and fruit. There was so much it was going bad before it could be eaten. For me, this just added to my stress. The waste sent me up a wall. Everyone thought it was so wonderful. I tried to be polite, but it was infuriating to see bags of food just going to waste. The final straw was when a group came over one day to clean. Don't get me wrong; they did a good job cleaning, but I couldn't find a thing after they left. I would spend more time trying to find where a dish or pan was put than it took to cook the meal. Clothes were put in the wrong closets, socks were mismatched, washcloths and towels were in the wrong place—the house was a tidy disaster from an organizational standpoint. At the time, we were spending a great deal of time in hospitals, so I wasn't paying much attention to detail. But once we were home and I had to do things for Annette, it was extremely difficult to do the simplest things. The entire house was in an uproar.

Then there was family. For weeks on end, they were practically living at our house. All day long someone was there—sometimes two or three at a time. Just imagine, from the time you got up until the time you went to bed, other people outside of your immediate family were in your home looking for something that needed to be done. And when the chores were completed, all they wanted to do was talk about your wife's condition. What did the doctor say? How long will the treatment take? How is she feeling? And on and on and on. Never in a group, but individually, as they arrived. In between that were the phone calls with the same inquiries. It was maddening. My wife was extremely ill, teetering on the edge of death. I just wanted to be alone. I needed time to think and cry and try to put some sense of logic to this entire mess. I realize that it was all done with the best of intentions, but the simple fact remained: it was adding to my stress level, not relieving it. I see now how close I was to going over the edge. This frustration had been building now for close to two months, and I just couldn't take it anymore. I know Annette liked having her family there, but she wasn't the one dealing with them.

I started taking control. First, I changed the message on our answering machine to say, "Hello, this is Rocco. If you are calling to chitchat, don't leave a message. If it is important, leave your name." (Note, I didn't say anything about a number. If you were a player, I already had your number. If I didn't have a number, then you were outside the loop, and I didn't care what you had to say.) Then I finished with, "If you are looking for information about Annette, consider no news as no changes."

We also set up a system using the e-mail. Originally, Kim was the official contact for Annette's friends, and John ran a site for our other friends and relatives. If you recall, Kim and Mike had a fire in their home. The same day that I called to tell them that Annette was diagnosed with cancer for the second time. Oddly enough, it worked out well. For the week that we were at Kensington Hospital, Kim and her family moved in to our house. This way they had a home while the insurance company was setting up accommodations for them, and we had someone that would be able to take care of the boys. This is what some people refer to as a mixed blessing. Some blessing. One person gets cancer, and an entire family is forced from their home. Where is the blessing? Next time, if it's alright with you, I'll pass. At this point, all of the addresses that Kim had were sent to John, and he became the official source of information regarding Annette's condition. Not only did he get the facts directly from Bill or me, but I could control what was being released. As I mentioned before, Annette's condition had a way of changing as the wind blew, so I didn't want every little detail to get out—only the information that we knew to be constant. This was very helpful in cutting down the phone calls and eliminating the rumors.

The next thing we addressed (which, by the way, was done through the e-mail) was visitation. It was getting way out of control. People were coming without notice one on top of the other. I was getting ready to install a revolving door. We decided the only way of keeping a handle on visits so Annette could get some rest was to get the word out that anyone wanting to come visit needed to call ahead and make sure it was a good time. This also would save them a trip, because I had gotten to the point that I didn't care who it was—if Annette wasn't up to the visit, then they weren't coming in. We also noted on the site that they needed to keep their visit to fifteen minutes. All visits had to include as many people as possible. For example, if six of her friends wanted to visit, they had to do their best to try and coordinate a time and day. So instead of six individual visits, which Annette couldn't tolerate anyway, She would get one or two visits with multiple visitors. This made it more fun, and it was easier on Annette. We were also able to fill them in on the latest without repeating ourselves all day long. It worked out very well, and everyone did the best they could to accommodate us.

One such visit came just after Christmas. About seven of her friends got together to visit one day. They were sitting in the family room. Most everyone was sitting on the floor in a half circle around the couch where Annette was lying down. They were having a wonderful time talking and laughing when, all of a sudden, I hear a scream followed by a roar of laughter. I was in the kitchen at the time doing dishes. I ran to the family room to see what was up. I couldn't believe my eyes. Annette was kneeling on the couch looking out the window into the backyard, just laughing to beat the band. This was the first time in about a month and a half that she had even sat up, let alone kneel and laugh. As it turned out, two of her friends got dressed up in overcoats with their bra and panties on the outside of their clothing and were dancing a jig in the backyard all while wearing antlers and a moose hat on their heads. I had to admit, it was quite a sight.

I know I was venting here a little, so I want to make it very clear. Annette and I were and still are extremely grateful for all of the help and support we received from our families, friends, and the community in general. There is no doubt that the love and compassion that all of you have expressed through your kind words and actions are truly a blessing. I hope and pray that not any of us will have to experience this again, but if we do, please remember the best support you can give to those in need begins with organization.

Faith

When I was in tenth grade, I had a steady girlfriend. Her name was Michelle. Well, as things go in high school, there was a dance one Friday night, and Michelle couldn't go, so I decided to go by myself with a couple of buddies. That night, I met a girl. She was new to the school and, quite frankly, I don't even remember her name now, but we spent the entire evening together. I had a wonderful time. I was on cloud nine until I got home and went to bed, and then all I could think about was, what am I going to tell Michelle? She's going to ask how the dance was. She expected me to dance with a couple girls during the dance but not spend the entire time with one girl. There was no use in trying to lie about it, because I lived in a very small town. Heck, my graduating class was eighty-seven students. As you all remember, your life revolved around the events of the school day. I was distraught, and I couldn't shake it. I really didn't do anything wrong. I didn't even kiss her. All we did was dance and talk, and I felt like I ruined my life forever. Later that night while lying in bed, I prayed for relief. I made a promise to God never to get into that situation again. I promised to do a lot of things that night (except become a priest) if only God would grant me peace. And it came. In an instant, I felt this overwhelming sensation of comfort come over me. It was something that I never experienced before in my life, and I knew that it wasn't of this world. Since that day, I have believed in a greater power. I believed in God. At least I thought I did. You may think this is a little extreme and I agree with you but I was young and this was my first serious relationship, my world revolved around Michelle. I was a kid in high school. You remember those days, everything was a major issue. What did I know.

Over the years, as life goes on, there are times in your life that make you wonder and question your beliefs. I always seemed to return back to the church and, in many cases, I came back with a stronger faith. If you were to ask me today, I would have to say that I don't know. I don't know if there is a God. This latest chapter in my life has taxed my beliefs beyond the edge. My belief in God is shattered; I don't know how I will recover from it this time. In the past, I found comfort in the community of our parish, and now it scares me to think that I lost that spiritual tie.

I do believe that at some point in history a man named Jesus—a very profound individual with an insight into human nature that has yet to be challenged—walked the earth. Was he the son of God? Or was he an extremely wise scholar? I don't know, but I do know that I believe in what he was trying to teach us, and I work very hard at living my life by his teachings.

There is a lot of hypocrisy out there when it comes to religious beliefs. Or should I say, there is some hypocrisy in the way some "religious" people live their lives. They claim to be children of God. They claim to be Christians and feel they are generous and caring. Some of these individuals believe they are companionate—just don't try and change lanes in front of them on the expressway. Or they somehow justify it being OK to steal the salt and pepper shakers from a restaurant or hack through the internet to access areas that will provide them a service free of charge. Then there are those who feel it is OK to steal from the company they work for. Why not? They can afford it, right? Besides, it's not stealing when you take from a faceless corporation. The logic makes my head spin.

I used to work with a guy that claimed to be very religious. He was very active in his church and even drove the church bus on Sunday. I guess he felt that he only had to follow the teachings of the church on Sunday, because during the week he didn't hesitate to charge people for parts that they didn't need when repairing their equipment. I have to tell you, he doesn't work for that company anymore. People just don't realize that when the cashier gives you that extra dollar in change and you knowingly put it in your pocket and walk away, that you just stole that dollar. Annette and I have tried to teach our boys that it's not only what you believe but how you incorporate your beliefs into your life that make you what you are.

When Annette became ill, many of her friends and family came running to her side with their bibles and prayer books and tapes and music in hand. They prayed over her with song and scripture.

In the beginning, when the doctors thought Annette had an infection, one of her friends happened to be at the hospital when it was discovered that Annette's PICC line plugged up. Annette was scheduled to go home that day, it was thanksgiving and she really wanted to be at home for the holiday. The first attempt to clear the line failed. So the nurse left to get a flush. A flush is nothing more than a heprin solution that is injected into the line to break down any build up and clear the passage. While the nurse was away getting the necessary supplies, this friend began her ritual of prayer and song and was thoroughly convinced that God would intercede and unplug the line before the nurse returned with her equipment. Although I felt that this was a bit extreme, I didn't say anything. I guess I wanted to see for myself. When the nurse returned, Annette's friend convinced her to try again before she infused the solution that she had gone to get. Well, it didn't work; Annette's line was still plugged. Our friend was disappointed, to say the least. She just couldn't believe that she called on God, and he didn't respond.

I wonder sometimes, Did they come to pray for Annette's healing, or did they come looking for some kind of sign to confirm that God is real? I wonder this because some have stopped coming. I realize that these people came with hope in their hearts and cures in their hands out of love and compassion, and maybe they stopped coming because they realized it may be making matters worse. But they never relayed that to me, so I guess I will never know the answer.

Let me say that everyone that came with a possible miracle called in advance and asked permission to come. I never refused anyone—how could I? What was I to say, no? We tried everything that was available, regardless of its nature or probability of a successful outcome. We were desperate, and amongst the desperation the fact that each failure only brought Annette's spirit down eluded me. Every time someone came with water or oil and it didn't work, it would bring down Annette's spirit. Think about it as if you were trying to save a friend from quicksand, and each time you reached out with a rope or a branch you prayed, "May God's love give strength to this branch, so as to be strong enough to save my friend," and it broke anyway!! With each effort, the person sank a little deeper and lost a little more hope, so what good have you done?

If you are ever in this situation where the person that is ill has a strong faith, I suggest that you bless them with the oil or water while they are sleeping; this way, if it doesn't work, they won't be the wiser. And if they do receive a miracle, you can tell them after the fact what you did. I don't think God would hold back a miracle just because the recipient is sleeping or unaware of your gift. If it is to be, it will be.

Like anything else in life, there are those that come to your side and stay regardless of the outcome. Annette's mother, sisters, and brother, along with her closest friends, never wavered. Their love and support gave Annette the strength to endure as long as she did. I thank all of you for that. I could take care of her medication and keep her warm and clean, but all of you gave her the love and hope she needed to keep fighting. You kept her faith, hope, and spirit alive. I thank you from the depths of my soul for all your strength and caring.

One person made a chart that was divided up into fifteen-minute increments so as to create a twenty-four-hour prayer chain. We had people praying all over the world for Annette's recovery. I do mean that literally. A few days after the chain was started, a phone call came from a friend of Kim's in England. Because of the difference in time, they offered to take the late-night hours of the chain. So they gathered friends of theirs and passed on their names to be added to the board. They don't know Annette; all they know is that a friend of Mike and Kim's was in a fight for her life, and they wanted to help. The humanity and compassion of their action was what I truly believe Jesus was trying to teach us. Every time I think of those people my eyes begin to well up with tears. This is what joins the soul. This is what connects all of us to the spirit.

It's funny how my belief in an almighty god has wavered. But I have an unwavering belief in angels, and I believe that when you die you go on to a different world, a different state of existence.

Here is an interesting story. People ask, "How can you believe in angels but not in God? Well, I start by reminding them that it's not that I don't believe in God. My belief is wavering right now. My belief in angels comes from a personal experience that I had last year. One night, a little over a year before Annette became ill, I had the strangest feeling that someone was in our bedroom. You know the feeling when the hair on the back of your neck stands up, your heart starts pumping, and you can feel the adrenaline flowing? I had that feeling the night before Annette caught a bad case of pneumonia. I was lying on my right side facing Annette. Without moving a muscle, I slowly opened my left eye to see if I could see anyone else in the room. To my amazement, I saw a small child sitting on Annette's dresser. I know I wasn't dreaming; I was fully awake by this time. I watched for a few seconds trying to focus in on this child. When I moved my head slightly to get a better look, the angel disappeared. I went from a heightened state of defense to complete calm in a few short seconds. The next morning, I told Annette what I saw. I'm not sure if she believed me or not, but when she was in bed for four weeks with pneumonia, I assured her that she would be alright.

"How do you know?" she asked.

I brushed back her hair and said, "Because of the angel I had seen. I know that angel is here looking over you right now."

She took my hand placed it on her chest. "Do you feel my heart beating?"

"Yes, why?" I asked.

"I want you to feel the love I have for you as it is being pumped through my body. If I have an angel," she said, "it is because of your love for me that has brought it here." Then she reached up with her other hand and pulled me close. That kiss will be one that I will always remember.

I have learned of prayers being said all over the country. It seems that everyone and anyone has taken the time to call a friend to have prayers said for Annette. Someone told me that they told their cousin, and that person told an in-law, and that person told a friend that lives in California who then included Annette in their prayers at church. The whole world is praying for my wife, and yet there still is no response; she continues to suffer daily. If there is a god, where is he or she? My wife's belief and lifestyle has influenced so many people, and Annette has touched so many lives that they are praying for her all over the world, yet for the last five months she has suffered every single day. I'm not just talking ill. Annette is violently ill. She will have episodes of vomiting that get so intense that you can hear the tendons and the joints of her bones popping from the stress. Her entire body tremors as if she is having a seizure.

I can understand illness and death—it is part of life, and there is nothing you can do about it. Children die of disease. People die in automobile accidents and plane crashes. Some are stricken with paralysis and other inflictions. I weep for those who have lost a family member or friend prematurely or unexpectedly. I'm angered for all who have to endure the suffering. I don't understand the reason. Is it not bad enough that they have been inflicted with a debilitating disease that prevents them from enjoying some of the simplest pleasures of life such as breathing? Why do they have to feel it every minute of every day? I'm so angry right now. I just don't understand why Annette has to suffer every single minute of every single day. She has never abandoned God—why has he abandoned her? She has cancer and will probably die from it—OK, we can deal with that. Please tell me why she has to be reminded of it continually. Can someone please tell me the reason why she has to feel it every waking moment? I'm down on my knees pleading to you to explain to me why the suffering exists. It's not self-inflicted, and no one is standing over her hitting her with a bat or prodding her with a knife. Her own body is creating these indescribable pains. This is what I don't understand. Why does He allow the suffering? What happened to the compassion, the humanity? The Bible teaches that we are put here on this earth to help our fellow man, to be there and protect those who cannot protect themselves. Why won't he step in and protect Annette?

Friends have said, "You have to hang in there. He is an 'eleventh-hour God.' Just when you feel you can't go any further, he steps in to comfort you." Isn't that just what she needs, a John Wayne God! Others have told me, "You must have faith. He must have a purpose, and he is using Annette because she is so strong, and he knows she will endure." It seems to me the kings of the dark ages used that same philosophy in their torture chambers to control the peasants. What message is God possibly sending that would require one person to endure such agony month after month, day after day, hour after hour, minute after minute, second after second?

When I was growing up, there was a bully in the neighborhood that would capture one of us and twist our arm until the rest of us gave up our lunch money. And if we hesitated, he would just twist harder and longer. I refuse to believe that God is a bully. And I don't understand how anyone could think that this is some form of message.

Then there's the old standby, "Just keep praying, and he will come." Well, you know what? If Annette has to beg minute after minute, and her friends and family have to beg and plead day after day for relief, well, for Annette's sake . . . I won't tell you what I feel right now about God.

Many people have advice. Most of it is a crock. At first, I was allowing it to add to my stress. Finally, I decided to only listen to advice from someone if they were willing to come and spend an entire twenty-four-hour day with Annette and then see if they could come up with some profound reason why her guts are being ripped out of her and then put back so she can do it again twenty minutes later.

Annette's faith, unlike mine, never wavered, and she never hesitated to admit her faith. There are quite a few people out there that say they believe, but when a situation comes up that puts them in a position that contradicts the teachings of their belief, they coward under peer pressure and stand by while things are said or done that they know in their hearts to be wrong. Annette lived by His word, speaking up when she felt things weren't right. Now she didn't get on a soapbox and preach chapter and verse from the Bible, but she made it clear that what was going on wasn't right. I cannot except that after the commitment she has made to her god that she still has to beg endlessly for help—help that has yet to come.

We were at Kensington Hospital when I was told that in order for prayers to be answered you have to be boisterous . . . give it all you've got. God doesn't answer a silent prayer. Essentially, I was being told that it was my fault that the prayers for Annette weren't being answered, because I prayed quietly in my own thoughts.

Isn't that a wonderful thing? Not only was my beloved wife being taken from me, but it was my fault that everyone else's prayers were in vain. I couldn't believe my ears. Those words cut through me like an old rusty steak knife, tearing and clawing at my inner soul. Later that evening, after everyone had gone home or to the hotel room, I began thinking about what I was told. I realized then that what that person said to me was out of grief and that she surely didn't mean it to come across the way it did. A lot of things were said in that room over the next few days that probably never would have been said, so I put it aside.

I did start to think about what she said, though, and thought that maybe I could try to do more. By this time, we had already been at this for over a month, and I was losing my faith fast. Then I thought, if I didn't believe at least somewhat in God, then how come I'm so mad at him? Do you see what I'm getting at? Only an insane person would be mad at someone that didn't exist. And Lord knows (an ironic phrase, don't you think, for someone who doesn't believe?) I'm as rational as the next guy. So I wrote a letter to God and put it up on the corkboard with all of the get-well cards. Here is the letter I wrote that night:

"Dear God,

It was explained to me by a priest that prayer isn't about asking for things, but about asking about things. Don't pray for yourself, pray for your neighbor, your family, your friends. Pray for those who can't help themselves. My prayer to you is, why do small children die? What good can come from the loss of parents, leaving orphans behind alone in the world? In our case, why must Annette endure such a "test"? She lives faithfully by your Word, always there to comfort the members or our community when they need help. She is so widely loved that thousands of prayers have been said, yet each day brings more bad news. Why must she beg for help? She has been faithful and loyal to your calling, and still she suffers. Not just physically but mentally. Two, joined together as one in your church, we didn't ask, why us?

This would mean we could accept this as a part of life as long as it happens to someone else. The anguish that we have endured should not be anyone's burden. My question to you is, why must the suffering exist at all? When you called on Peter to follow you, did you then ask him to do it without the use of his legs? Annette has heard your call and has touched the lives of many people. And now you want her to beg for her life so she can continue on. Well, that's not right in my book. Show her your love by showing her the light at the end of the tunnel. She will suffer and endure, but she needs to know you are there."

                                                                Rocco

I want to believe. Sometimes I feel it is easier to believe. When things get tough or when someone dies, it is easy to say, "It's God's will. He has a plan. It is not ours to question why." Those are easy things to say, but I'll bet they were never said by the people that were directly involved.

What kind of plan can justify the pain and suffering?

I question my faith now, and I believe that there are many others who have also questioned their faith when faced with such an impasse. I don't know where I will end up, but I do know that it will not affect how I continue to live my life. As I said before, I do believe that Jesus existed, and I truly believe that his teachings are the essentials for preserving your soul. If there is a god and if there is a heaven, I promise you now, if I make it to heaven, I will personally ask God why this ever had to come to be. If there is a plan or was a plan, I want to know the results, and I'm sure as heck going to find out how it was determined that this was the only method available. God or no God, this is my wife, the woman that I vowed to honor and protect in his church. How could God do this to his own his own child?

WOW!

This is an entirely new thought. All this time I was focused on Annette as my wife, not as one of his children. Oh my, who would put their own child through such agony and suffering? We lock those people up and throw away the key. But we accept this behavior from God?

I have to stop writing now. This is making my head spin. I am not a theologian, and the scope of that question alone could be a book in itself.

It has been awhile since I wrote that last paragraph, and I have had a lot of time to reflect and ponder the questions that have troubled me. It has occurred to me that there is no divine plan. Some ask me who am I to question God and His plan. I simply tell them that I'm not questioning God. I'm questioning those who tell me to accept Annette's suffering as some sort of divine plan.

Who are they to know? Did they go to God and say, "What's the deal? Show us the plan." You know the answer to that question.

The fact is, it is a rationalization—a rationalization that is thousands of years old. Well, if were going to rationalize, why not use some logic? This is my thought on the subject. Maybe I'm wrong and maybe I'm not, but I can live with my rationalization. My rationalization has given me peace and has allowed me the time and energy needed to comfort Annette.

Somehow it is an accepted practice to praise God for all the good things in this world, but the bad things are just written off as being part of the plan. If this was true, if this divine plan does exist; then God would have to sit there and say, "We need a mixture of good things and devastating things."

Oh wait, maybe he has a meeting with his cabinet of saints and asks, "What is our good-to-bad ratio?"

"Oops. Things are going too good. We had better throw in a few natural disasters, and let's raise the infant fatality rate by 10 percent and throw in another psychopath leader. We haven't had one of those for about sixty years."

"Yeah! Remember Hitler?" a cabinet member says.

"Ooh, man. He was a good one," God says.

"Well we have Saddam", voices another cabinet member.

"Yeah but Hitler ruled the charts". God says

I DON'T THINK SO!!!!!!

If there is a divine plan, then that's how it has to be. All the celebration, peace, joy, disasters, murders, wife beaters, child molesters, rapists, suffering, pain, and on and on and on, have to be planned out. I cannot accept that god plans out a disaster that takes thousands of lives. Or figures in a rapist, murderer into the mix for variety.

If God is a loving God, then it doesn't fit. Ask any builder, architect, or organizer this question. If you only have a partial plan, can you begin, let alone complete, a project? Do you think an architect takes the time to draw up a complete set of plans with everything planned out to the finest detail and then turns it over to the builder and say, "Here is the blueprint. And, oh, by the way, you have the right of choice. You can deviate from the blueprint wherever you please."

God is perfect, right? That's what we've all been taught. I just can't see a perfect God that created a world with an imperfect plan. So, you see, either there is a plan or there isn't. I'm darn sure there isn't a partial plan.

I was told that the suffering is part of the plan, because Jesus suffered on the cross. A statement like that can only come from someone that has never watched a loved one suffer, I'm not talking from a far where you stop in occasionally to visit or call to see how things are going. I'm talking about being in the trenches 24 hours a day. I'm also not talking about watching a parent, sibling or friend, even though that can be a close relationship. It is not the same as watching your spouse or your child be torn apart relentlessly. The question is, was it Gods plan for his son or your spouse or your child to be brutally tortured until they died? It was Gods plan to have nails driven through Jesus' hands and feet after being whipped and tortured? Or was that merely the act of his aggressors? I refuse to believe that God planned for his son to be viciously murdered. It was the Romans decision to nail Jesus to the cross not Gods plan. God gave us the freedom to choose and that is what they did. I do believe that God reached down at that moment to comfort his son in his time of need.

We have all heard the saying "God helps those who help themselves" I understand that statement now more than ever before. It is my belief that God knows each individuals strengths and weaknesses. Based on your efforts to build your character, God presents to you opportunity. What ever opportunities you have been given, you have earned them, based on the effort you have put into living a good and productive life. It is up to you, it is your choice whether you seize that opportunity or let it pass by. This doesn't mean that these opportunities come without struggles, for it is the struggles and challenges in life that build the foundation of your character.

And don't give me this business about the devil or Satin or the beast or whatever it is you want to call temptation; as the reason why people do bad things to themselves or others. Temptation is merely an excuse for the weak of heart. Do we all give in to temptation; you're darn right we do. Lets just point the finger in the direction it belongs.

I believe that when God set things in motion he had a choice to make. "Do I give them the ability to make decisions, to choose between right and wrong, or do I plan out every little detail? If I create a plan and lay out every detail, then my children won't be living, they will merely exist. On the other hand, if I give them the ability to choose, then I cannot control life, and there will be uncertainty, happiness, joy, pain, suffering, and peace, all intermingled. Some will live long lives, and some will not. Some will choose right, and some won't. Some will suffer, and some won't.

"BUT! (And this is a big but.) I can be there to comfort them and guide them through the bad times. They will live. My children will experience the beauty of being alive."

I believe God's plan is not to have a plan, but to give us opportunity, guidelines and support.

This makes much more sense to me than a god that could put a three-year-old child or my wife through the agony of cancer. Or create murders and rape. Not only allow it to happen, but to actually plan it out. And if there is a divine plan, then we have to accept the fact that God could do this to his own children. You cannot have it both ways. I can accept the fact that he gave us the right of choice, and that package came with the uncertainty of life.

I cannot believe there is a divine plan that contains all of the pain and suffering. If there is a plan, and in that plan everyone had a set time to die, why does it have to involve suffering and pain? He's God. He can harvest souls anytime, PEACEFULLY!

I just don't buy the divine-plan theory. God is a loving God. He gave us the freedom to choose. And like any good father, he lets his children find their own way, giving support and love along the way. If I'm going to believe in God, it has to be this way.

The last time Annette was in the hospital, I awoke around 1:00 a.m. and wrote the following letter to her. (I placed it at this point in the book because this is what opened my eyes and my heart. These thoughts allowed me to come to terms with Annette's illness.)

Dear Annette,

When you first became ill, you had me grab this spiral pad to keep a record of your medication and treatments. Who would have thought I would use all but these last few pages? This book is not only a record of all you have been through, but a testimony to our life together. In these last five months, we have lived a lifetime of emotions through your suffering and strength.

For twenty years, you have been by my side, never once second-guessing the decisions we made or our life together.
When I proposed to you, I said, "Come with me. I make 400 dollars a month, and we're going to live in the desert 2000 miles from home."

And you said, "OK!"

I said, "Come with me. Let's go to Lake Mead in my boat. It only leaks a little."

And you said, "OK."

You went to the store one day, only to find the kitchen wall torn out when you returned. I looked at you and said, "Let's remodel the kitchen."

And you said, "OK."

I was between jobs when I came to you and said, "Let's start a family."

And you said, "OK."

In November, you came to me and said, "I have a long journey to travel. Come be by my side."

And I said, "OK."

For the longest time I couldn't understand how God could allow you to suffer for so long. Then I realized that it wasn't God; it was you. You were fighting the violent pain, not for yourself, but for the boys and me, for your mother and sisters and brother, for all your family and friends. So we could have time to say good-bye. So we would have time to say all that needed to be said. So we could prepare for life without you.

Then, once again, God called to you. "Annette, come with me." You turned from the light and looked all around.

Then you turned back to God

and said, "OK."

As on our wedding day, before all these witnesses I proclaim my eternal love. You are in my heart and in my soul. One day we will be together again. Please wait for me.

"OK."

Love,
Rocco

I had John read this as part of Annette's eulogy. To give you an idea of the impact Annette had on the lives of the people of our community, over five hundred people paid their respects at the funeral home, and a little over three hundred people attended her service.

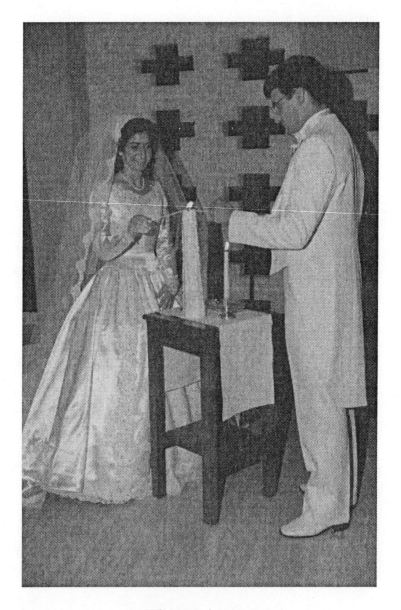

When two became one

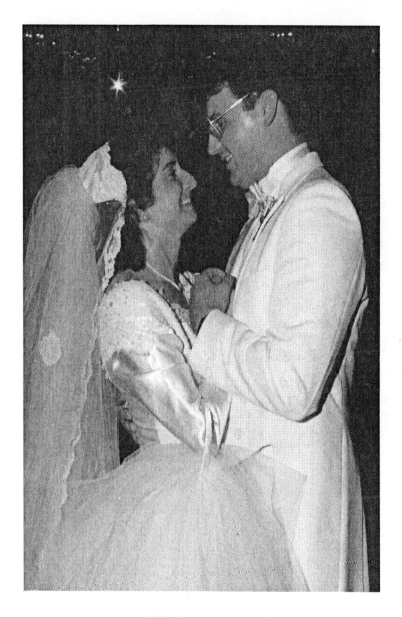

This dance never ended

Chapter 4

Grieving

All wedding ceremonies include an exchange of vows that both the bride and groom proclaim to each other. Some write their own vows, and some use the old standby. The one thing they all have in common is that they end with "till death do us part." Would you like some inside information? It doesn't end with death. The love and commitment continues on. They say the stronger and deeper your love for each other, the stronger and more agonizing the grieving is—and they are right.

The grieving process will begin and end differently for each individual. In my case, my grieving began the night Annette became ill. Her pain was so intense that between the pain and the medication to fight it, she had lost all of her desire for carrying on our relationship as we knew it.

Let me explain what I mean. Annette loved me dearly; in fact, as things went along, our love grew even stronger. But the day-to-day romance was gone. This is a common event. It happens to every one of us from time to time, only you don't realize it, because it is only a temporary breach. Think of the last time you were very ill. Did you love your spouse any less? The answer is no, you loved your spouse just as much. Chances are, you gained a greater appreciation for them, because they were caring for you, but you had no desire for romance. All you wanted to do was lie there and get better. Because it is short-term, the absence of affection is not missed.

The night Annette became ill, was the moment that our life together, as we knew it, changed forever. Imagine that, without warning, all romance and physical affection was removed from your marriage in one brief moment. That's what happened to our relationship. Except for a handful of times over the next five months, never again would I be the recipient of a smile that was wrapped in desire. We would never dance together or carry on a conversation that didn't involve medical treatments. Her desire to touch me and caress my body was gone. For the next five months, I would share a bed with her, never to make love again or to even cuddle up next to her because of the physical pain it would cause. Rarely was I able to hold her or even touch her skin without causing pain or nausea. As the time grew, the despair grew. I was starved for affection. I wanted so bad to ravish her with love and be ravished by her.

I became so desperate for her affection that one day I created a scenario that, under normal circumstances, would have sparked her desire. When Annette was still able to walk, I set up a stool in the shower and asked if she would prefer a shower instead of a bath. The thought was if we were both in the shower she would be aroused enough to at least reach out and touch me. All I wanted was a touch. All I wanted was to have her show me some form of desire. I knew it was in there; I knew she carried it with her. I needed to find a way that would stimulate her passion so great that it would emerge from the depths with all the force and glory that you see when a whale surfaces from the ocean floor. I was so desperate for affection I stooped to an adolescent trick such as this. It didn't work. The desire was buried, consumed by pain and masked in a cloud of medication. Annette just sat there as I washed her body. Not a single remark. She didn't smile, not even a wink. Never again would we share our life of physical passion.

Again, it's not that she didn't want to. In my soul, I know she still wanted me; it was the pain and the medication that had dulled her senses. I knew then that I would never again know the feeling of Annette's desire for my love. All I could do was watch her slowly die. Regardless of all of the care and medicine, I wouldn't be able to stop it.

At the time I didn't realize it, but this is when my grieving began. I had to ignore it in order to care for her. But it was there waiting in the lurch, growing stronger by the day until a day or two after Annette's funeral, when it came pouring through.

131

Booze and Drugs

The beginning of the grieving process is a very critical time. This is the time that you are the most vulnerable. Drugs and alcohol become very attractive devices to help deaden the pain. Unfortunately, there are some that can never pull themselves out of the bottle once they have fallen into it. You must remember this next statement. Cut it out if you have to, enlarge it, and mount it on the walls of your home. DRUGS AND ALCOHOL **ARE NOT, ARE NOT, ARE NOT** THE ANSWER. They will numb your senses, yes, but they will hinder, if not altogether, stop the grieving process. And if that happens, you will never, ever heal. If you don't heal, you will never live again.

I was fortunate. I was into the bottle at a rate of almost a fifth a day. (It didn't take me long to get there either. It had been less than a week after Annette died, and I didn't care that it was only 10:00 a.m.—I was hitting the bottle.) One day, John asked me if my consumption of alcohol had increased. (John uses words like that. "Consumption of alcohol." Anyone else would say, "Have you been hitting the bottle?") My brother Russ asked me that same question at the funeral home, but I lied to him.

One night about eight, John asked again about my "consumption." I told him that I was on my tenth drink of the day. Not only was I concealing the fact that the glass of coke was half soda and half booze, but my behavior didn't indicate that I had been drinking at all. That is, everyone thought I was just depressed, when, in fact, depression accounted for only a portion of my physical condition.

John packed up all of my booze and took it back home to Illinois with him. I gave my word to go one month booze-free, and I kept my word. I was very fortunate to have a friend that was looking at the big picture and had the courage to run interference. I would hate to think of where I would be if he hadn't stepped in.

Suicide

I'm going to enter this area with a great deal of caution. I say that because I'm not a crisis counselor, and I realize this is no place for amateurs. All I want to say is, I was there. I think anyone who lost a spouse they admired and loved with all of their heart and soul as I did Annette has contemplated suicide as a means of ending the pain. I remember the exact moment. It was one week to the day that John had put me on the wagon and two-and-a-half weeks since Annette died. I was getting ready for bed. I wasn't sleeping much then, and it wasn't uncommon for me to be up into the early morning hours. To this day, I can picture myself standing at the sink. My eyes were bloodshot, and my face was riddled with grief. Those were the days that I spent most of my time crying. Blowing out Annette's candle at the end of the day was good for at least a fifteen- or twenty-minute breakdown of tears and groans of pain. I remember looking into the mirror and thinking how easy it would be to just take the entire bottle of sleeping pills. Pouring them out in my hand and filling a cup of water. I was there. I was consumed by my own pain. My thoughts were riddled with ideas of escape that were accompanied with illogical conclusions. Ideas that I believed would reunite Annette and me. Ideas that would allow me to regain Annette's passion, a passion that I desperately desired. I was ready. I had convinced myself that this was the path to take. As I placed those pills in my mouth and began to raise that water to my lips, the dead of night was shattered when I heard my ten-year-old son, Jacob, yell out in his sleep, "What? What do you want?" His cry drove right to my soul. It snapped me out of the trance that was consuming my thoughts. The water glass flew from my hand, and pills landed everywhere as I spit them out. I curled up on the floor in a fetal position and sobbed until I fell asleep.

That was the night Annette saved my life.

You see, Jacob is a heavy sleeper and is extremely difficult to wake, but when you do, he always says, "What? What do you want?" before rolling over and going back to sleep. I know it was Annette stepping in. She was the one that roused Jake from his sleep in an attempt to reach me. When

I awoke, I sat there in amazement that I could have even contemplated suicide. I was terrified. How can grief take such a hold on your reasoning that you abandon all logical thought and allow it to guide your actions? I don't ever remember being so afraid of any one thing ever before. The ramifications would be disastrous. The greatest and most tragic of all the consequences that could sprout from this situation would have been the fact that my boys would be left to face this world alone. I would give my eternal soul to protect them—how could I even consider suicide? It was the grief. It was the pain. It horrifies me to think what I would have done if I had been drinking at the time.

Blame

A couple weeks after I sobered up, I began running and rerunning different scenarios that may have led to Annette getting cancer. It was maddening. You see, the one thing that I couldn't get over was that this all started after I procrastinated about removing some boxes from the car.

Let me explain. About three weeks before Annette became ill, I had purchased some brochure shelves for the office. There were three boxes, and they were extremely heavy. I should have taken them directly to the office, but it would have meant me fighting rush-hour traffic, and I wanted to go home. Well, the next day, Annette was going to pick up an air-hockey table that we had bought the boys for Christmas and drive it over to the shop to store it until Christmas Eve. I should have warned her about their weight, but I figured she would have the guys at the shop unload everything—the boxes and the hockey table. What I didn't count on and didn't even think of was at the store, when she picked up the air-hockey table. The boxes were in the way, and she couldn't fold the seat down. But instead of asking the stock boys at the store, she moved the boxes herself.

A couple days later, she had a terrible pain in her shoulder that wouldn't go away. She went to see Bill, and he gave her some medication along with instructions to take it easy for a few days. It took almost two weeks for the pain to go away. And it really never went away completely. I overheard Bill talking to someone else about a month after Annette died. He said that when she came in for the pain in her shoulder, it could have been a blood clot moving through her system. Maybe she bruised something inside when she moved the boxes. Couple that with this Factor 5 thing, and she may have had a clot causing the pain.

The guilt cut through me like a razor. All of this was caused because I was too lazy to deal with traffic. I was heading into a deep depression. I was convinced I killed Annette. Because I was too lazy, she suffered all of those months. I was at fault; everything would be fine today if I would have moved the boxes.

135

The boys and I started seeing a grief counselor through hospice the week after Annette's funeral. This is where we met Cindy. Standing about five feet tall with curly red hair, she always greets you with a bright smile upon her face and a comfort in her voice. Cindy has dedicated her profession to helping those of us who face a world of uncertainty. Through caring and hope she walks with many as they travel along the passage that leads them through the vast dense forest of grief.

It was about 3 months after Annette's death that Cindy could tell I was going deep, and I wasn't surfacing for air. Asking question after question, trying to hit on what was causing this deep depression. I finally explained to her the guilt I was feeling. My laziness was responsible for Annette's death.

The beauty of a good, and I stress the word **good**, counselor is that they can open your eyes and your mind to different perspectives. She started off by pointing out the fact that you cannot get cancer from lifting a box. Plain and simple, it's a medical fact: you cannot get cancer from lifting a box. Chances are the cancer was already there, already growing, already sowing its seeds. Yes, lifting the box may have caused the clot. But Annette didn't die from a blood clot; she died from cancer. Even if she did die from the clot, she had a rare disease that created the clots, and there was nothing you could have done about that. I still wasn't totally convinced.

That's when she asked, "Was Annette active?"

"Yes," I replied.

"OK," she said. Looking at me square in the eye, she asks, "What if one of the boys had left their bike in the way of the car, and in order for her to move it she would have had to lift it over her head. Would that be a difficult thing for her to do?"

"Yes," I said with a hesitation in my voice. Although she was fit, Annette wasn't very strong.

Cindy continued, "If that would have been the scenario, would you be blaming your son for leaving his bike in the way of the car?"

"No, I certainly wouldn't."

"OK then, you can't blame yourself. What happened was tragic, but you didn't do anything wrong. You have nothing to feel guilty about."

She was right. It still took about a week to work that through, but eventually I came to terms with the fact that moving the boxes may have brought the cancer and the Factor 5 thing to the surface, but it didn't cause the cancer, and I didn't kill my wife.

Get Help—You Can't Do It Alone

Getting proper counseling is extremely important. You may only go for a month or so, or you may go for a couple of years. It is important to go, though. You need to seek professional help—help that your friends, family, clergy, or associates cannot provide you. They can't provide it, because they don't get it. Unless they lost their spouse under the same circumstances that you have (i.e., same age, same family situation, same type of relationship) they won't understand what you are going through. Even today, Cindy will say, "I can't tell you I understand what you are experiencing, but I can tell you that over the years and of the hundreds of patients that I have seen, many have told me that they have experienced this or experienced that." And that is what a good grief counselor can do for you. They give to you their past experiences. This can't be fixed with a textbook. There are so many variables that come into play. Each individual and the relationship they shared will determine the time needed to heal and the path it will take.

Society's Expectations— Just Remember, They Don't Get It

Before I get into society's take on your situation, let me enlighten you on some of the things you're going to encounter. For the most part, your friends and family will not understand what you are experiencing, and that is fine; they can't. Now that you are where you are, you can look back and see that before you lost your spouse, before you were plunged into the abyss, you didn't "get it" either. And that is fine; that's understandable. It's when those who have not lived your experience come up to you and say they understand what you are going through. Those are the folks you need to separate yourself from as quickly as possible. They are the ones that will give you the most misinformation as to how you are supposed to act and feel.

I've had divorcees come up to me and say they understand. They don't have a clue. Yes, they have grieved a loss; I don't deny them that. But there are a few major factors that they have not even considered. The first is, if they have young children like I do, they aren't going it alone—at least not for the most part. They share custody, and both parents are there to make decisions about their kids' welfare. Their ex is not dead. All they have to do is pick up the phone, even if it's just to complian about something. I would give anything to have Annette back, even if it was to just disagree on something. And the biggest, most grandiose reason of all that they cannot understand is: THEY MADE THE DECISION TO SEPARATE AND DIVORCE. Whether they feel they were forced to divorce or if they felt there was no other option but to divorce, the fact remains, they made that decision to follow through. We, as a group, didn't choose to lose our greatest love. No one came to us and offered us an option. The person we cherished was taken from us. Our feelings and pain weren't even considered. So unless someone has experienced your loss, proceed with caution when the advice starts to come. And if they are all-knowing, kindly or abruptly tell them to go away, and you will call them when you are ready. I don't care how close of a friend they were before your tragedy or if they are a family member that thinks they are doing what's best for you, send them away. If you don't, it will create confusion and cause you to have more stress, more grief.

You will find that society has accepted certain time limits for you to grieve. They go like this: You should be back to work within a couple weeks. (Here's a kicker for you. Many corporations, hospitals included, give their employees three days to grieve and get back to work. The hospital administrators DON'T GET IT.) You should be willing to attend family functions and friendly get-togethers within one month. So, you should be happy and functional by the end of thirty days. But it is socially unacceptable to seek companionship until after a year has passed. (You should still be in mourning, completely functional and happy, but still in mourning. Guess what? Society, as a whole, DOESN'T GET IT.) Let me say this loud and clear. Our society is the most dysfunctional group of individuals that ever inhabited this planet. You will know when it is time to return to work. You will know when you are ready to be social again, and you will definitely know when you are ready for another companion.

Unlike someone who loses a spouse in an accident or some other tragic event where death is instantaneous, my experience came in different stages. In fact, it came in three distinct stages or, should I say, affected three distinct parts: marriage, death, and relationship. Each part has its own place on the timeline.

Annette passed from this world to the next on March 29, 2003. And that's all that happened that day. This day was a day of peace for Annette, and although I couldn't see it at the time, it was a day of peace for all of us that were left behind. We all knew how much Annette suffered, and as terrifying as it was to let her go, we had peace in our hearts knowing that she was free from the pain. We know she is amongst family and friends; there's comfort in that.

Our marriage didn't end that day. In my heart and soul I will always be married to her. I will always love her and cherish the time we shared. Never again will my heart carry only one flame. I will always cherish the wedding band she gave me. I will always wish her a good morning and tell her good night. Not a day will pass that I don't tell her that I love her. And if I do meet someone else to spend the rest of my days on this earth with, they will be kind and understanding with a great deal of compassion. I say this because they will have to accept this flame I carry for Annette. There is some baggage that comes with this package. It's not heavy, but it does take up some space.

As I mentioned before, our relationship ended five months before her passing. So when did the grieving begin? It began the day that we could no longer interact the way we had for the last twenty years. For me, the grieving began the day Annette could no longer show her affection the way she truly wanted to. Our relationship, the desire ended November 2, 2002, almost five months before she passed away. I guess what I'm trying to say is that timelines don't exist. We will all have to travel this journey at our own pace. Hopefully, the ones that are most important to us, those who are closest to us, will give us the space and time we need to heal.

Chapter 5

The Whole

We have all been asked or have asked someone, "Where's your better half?" Or, "How is your better half?" What I didn't realize until Annette became ill was she wasn't my better half. She was more than that—she was the half that made me whole. When we took our vows, part of the ceremony included an act where, as two separate individuals, we walked side by side, both of us carrying a lit candle to a larger candle, where together we joined our two flames into one as we lit the larger candle. That minute, our love was in its infancy, a seed that had been sown, wrapped in love, caring, and compassion. As that seed grew, trust and devotion developed, which enveloped the love, caring, and compassion that grew stronger and produced admiration and appreciation, which enveloped the love, caring, compassion, trust, and devotion that grew ever stronger until there was us. We were two that grew into one.

Just as an apple grows from a seed and becomes whole, it can only survive as long as the two halves remain together. When Annette died, I didn't lose my better half, I lost one half of the whole. If you leave the apple intact, attached to the tree, it will live its intended life. But if you pick that apple and lop off half, what happens to the other half? It turns brown, shrivels up, and dies.

What has died is the life we had together. We will no longer share a place in this world together as one.

Grief is about healing the wound. And the more intertwined your souls are, the greater the wound to heal.

Healing

Will I physically shrivel up and die? No, although there are times when I wish I would, so as to not to have to endure the pain. The pain is as real as if you were being slowly tortured. In the beginning, it never stops either. You can put it aside temporarily with distractions such as work or caring for your kids or taking care of the house. But the minute you let down your guard, it comes right back. And it comes back with a vengeance. Just as water that has been backed up by a dam, it rushes in with all its force looking to swallow you up. The hardest thing about it, is you have to let it. It will never go away until you allow the process to complete itself. Your body has to heal.

Do you think you could prevent your arm from healing if it were broken? No, you couldn't; your body is going to do what it has to in order to mend. You can disrupt the healing, in which case your arm may grow back crooked and lose some of the uses that it was once capable of. But it will heal and mend. The choice is yours. Either allow it to heal properly or not. It is the same with grief. Your body has to physically and mentally mend. You can allow it to do so, or you can interrupt the process, in which case you may not function with the same capabilities as you did before.

The Process

Grieving is having two buckets, one bucket of good, and the other is a bucket of bad. When you start out, the good bucket is empty, and the bad bucket is filled to the brim. Keep in mind that the name on the bucket does not represent what is in them. It merely represents the level you are at when it comes to dealing with those items. For example the items that are in the bad bucket are not the things that were necessarily bad in your relationship. The items that will remain in the bad bucket are the things that are too difficult or too painful for you to remember or recall. For example, Annette and I went to Las Vegas twice a year. It was our time away from everything else; a time when we could sleep in as long as we wanted. We could go for an early morning walk for exercise or a late night stroll through a garden of flowers and fountains where we could stop and kiss along the way. It was a time that we could make love any time of the day that pleased us. When Annette and I went on these trips, we did many things such as playing pokers at the Mirage or going to watch a movie at the Orleans. Mostly though, these trips were for romance, they were the Super Bowl, World Series and Stanley Cup of our relationship. It was the time we shared, just the two of us to feed the fire of our desire for each other. I have been invited many times to fly out there for a few days; the one time I went I was miserable the entire trip. Vacationing in Las Vegas may very well remain in my bad bucket. I hope not because I really enjoyed going there. But as for now that is where it stays, in the bad bucket.

Being able to get through grieving isn't about filling the good bucket and emptying the bad; it's about balancing them out. You will never completely fill the good or empty the bad. The best you can do is to find a balance between them that will allow you to move on and live life happily, once again.

At first the bucket of bad has everything in it—everything you shared, agreed on, disagreed on, things you did, things you said, things that were special to you, and the million things that will never be again. Grieving is the process of sorting, sorting out the things that can be moved from the bad bucket to the good bucket.

The things that can be moved, over time, are the memories you shared. In the beginning, every thought, every recollection, will bring tears of sorrow and pain. As time passes, and each time you recall those memories, you will expose them and the emotions that accompany them, so your body can work through the healing—until the time comes when you recall that memory and realize that you aren't crying but smiling. It is at this time that you have successfully moved that one memory from the bad bucket to the good bucket. Some things are easier to move than others, but it seems that once you begin to transfer over some memories, it becomes easier to move more and more items over. I will warn you, though, in the beginning, those first few memories that get moved over to the good bucket come with a feeling of guilt. Guilt that after all those months of pain and agony you are moving on. DO NOT mistake this as casting aside the one you loved so deeply. You are merely coming to terms with the fact that your life has changed and it will never be the same again. You must remember, you are still here, and in order to live again, you have to move on. I know deep in my soul that Annette would want me to move on and enjoy life once again, and the only way to do this is to accept the fact that I cannot change what has happened.

When you are faced with a situation of this magnitude, your family and friends have a tendency to dig up all sorts of articles, poems, books, and little messages on cards, all in an effort to comfort you. Some are sent for what they are, words of encouragement and support to help you keep your spirit and hopes up, to let you know that you are not alone and that they are there if you need them. Others are sent with the idea that they are going to solve all of your problems in an instant, and life is going to be one big happy place again. Simply disregard the foolish attempt from people who obviously have a specific agenda. This agenda is not to help you heal, but to have you appear to be all better so they can feel better. It is a selfish act on their part, and you need to separate yourself from these distractions as quickly as possible. Your only concern should be your healing. I don't advocate selfishness, and I'm not saying that for the rest of your life you can expect everything to be me, me, me. But, for the time being, until you work through your grief, that is where your focus needs to be.

The hardest things to deal with are the "nevers." These will always be in the bad bucket. These are the things that we will never share again. I'll never glance across a room and see her beautiful smile as she winks at me. I'll never feel her skin pressed up against mine or be able to brush the back of my hand across her bottom as we pass in a crowded room. Never again will we go to one of our son's hockey games, hold hands as we walk on a cool spring night, make a holiday dinner together or share a date night. We will never again be able to look into each other's eyes and say "I love you." I'll never hold her hand, sit next to her on a plane, share a meal, hold her close and dance a slow dance, plan a vacation, decide what to have for dinner, or make love to her ever again. There are a million nevers. A million little details that I will never share with her again.

Date nights were mini vacations for us, they were filler times between our weekends away that we so dearly loved to do. These nights were quite simple in design; yet they were a staple on our list of items that fueled the romance in our relationship. A date night consisted of getting the boys to bed, we would then shower and get cleaned up just as if we were going out—only the farthest we ever went was to bed. With candles lit and soft music in the background, we would give each other a massage, talk about our dreams and share an intimate evening together.

The grieving process takes as long as it takes. Depending on the level of your relationship and what you shared will determine how long it takes you to begin transferring items from the bad bucket to the good bucket, and you may never finish the process. The point is, listen to your body; it knows you better than you think. It knows what you need to do to become physically and mentally healthy again.

Signs

Be open to experiences that seem out of the ordinary. They may come in the form of a dream or you may hear things around the house. For example; shortly after my dad died, my mother moved from the old farmhouse that they shared for over thirty years in to her new house near my brother. I remember her telling me that she would hear something tapping on the glass. After a week or so she said, "Ray, if that's you, just come on in." After that, she didn't hear the tapping anymore.

My own experience—well, the first one anyway—came a couple months after Annette died. One night I experienced that same feeling that I had the night the angel came and sat on Annette's dresser. The hair on my neck stood up, my heart started pounding, and the adrenaline was racing through my veins. As I did that night, I slowly opened one eye, but I didn't see anything this time. What I felt was unbelievable. All of a sudden, I could feel this warm sensation across my back and shoulders. It was indescribably comforting. A peaceful calm came over me; I could feel it travel through my entire body. After a moment, I rolled over to Annette's side of the bed, and I could smell her scent. Yes, I could smell her scent. Annette had this subtle scent that was only present right after she showered. It was the scent I had smelled a hundred times before when we would have our date nights. It was Annette who came to visit me that night. It wasn't until morning that I realized that the warm sensation I felt was her body next to mine. You know that warmth you feel when you lie next to someone, when there is no clothing to interfere with each other's skin touching? That kind of closeness carries soothing warmth that transfers from your partner to you. That is what I experienced that night. It was then I knew that Annette was with me. She may pop in and out from time to time, but I'm sure she stops in to check on us in between parties or picnics or whatever else they have going on over on the other side. She was a little socialite in this world; I'm sure she's the party planner on the other side. And that is a very peaceful feeling for me.

I mentioned before about the penny business. The boys, family, and friends seem to find them all over the place. I have only found one. I always said, it only counts if the coin is shiny and new. It has to be. If the coin you find is old and discolored, it has probably been there longer than Annette has been gone, so it can't be from her. The one I found was at a family reunion. It was getting late in the day, and I was getting tired, so I went and sat down at one of the tables. I had been sitting there for about fifteen minutes, my head was down, and I was just looking around under the table thinking about how much I missed her when my cousin came over and began to talk. I was a little teary, so she asked if I was OK. I raised my head and said, "Yeah. I was just thinking of Annette, wishing she was here." When I lowered my head again, lying there right in front of me on the cement pad was a shiny, new 2003 dime. I had been staring at that spot for fifteen minutes before that, and there was no dime there before. Just as we lived our lives, her messages aren't massive in quantity or lavish in cost. But they are always there at the right time, abounding with love.

Before I get to the best and most entertaining story, let me tell you about the sign I received from her dad. Annette's dad died ten months, almost to the day, before Annette died. After her dad died, whenever the boys found a penny, Annette would tell them, "That's Papa letting you know he is with you." As with Annette's coin, I always contended that they have to be shiny and new. Well, one night I was returning from a business trip in Chicago when I pulled over for gas. I stepped out of the car, slid my card in for payment, and started pumping gas into the tank. While I stood there killing time, I was looking all around as we all do. BUT, when I went to put the nozzle back on the rack, I spotted this brand-new shiny penny sitting on top of this pile of dirty, oil-ridden slush. When I bent over to pick up the penny, I noticed a screw lying a few inches away—then another and another. In all, I picked up twenty-three nails and screws that were scattered around my tires and under my car. I don't know how I missed them when I pulled in, but I'm sure I would have picked one or two up in my tires when I pulled away. Annette was between her first and second rounds of chemo at that time. So I brought them home and told her the story. Then I asked her, "Do you remember when you had pneumonia last year and an angel came to be with you?" She nodded. "Well, this time, your dad is here with you. Tonight was his sign to me, to let me know that he is here with you." She smiled and began to cry. I still have that bag of screws.

OK, let's lighten things up a bit. This is my favorite story, by the way.

Most cars today are designed to automatically lock the doors when the vehicle is put into drive or after they reach a certain rpm or rate of speed. Our van does not, I repeat, does not have this feature. It was a habit of Annette's to bring a bag of things to do in the car if we were going farther than the local store. Whenever we left the driveway, she would get settled in, and within the first mile, she would lock the doors. Well, about two months after she passed, the locks in the van would lock by themselves. Not all the time, but often enough for it not to be a fluke. Since then, whenever the doors lock, I know she is with me, and we have a nice conversation. It's funny, though. Now that I think about it, they usually lock whenever I'm mulling over a decision. Here is the kicker. On July 2, two days before we were to leave for a holiday weekend, a carload of kids came through the neighborhood shooting out car windows. And, yes, we were one of the victims. Not having a lot of time before leaving for a ten-day getaway, I went to the first place I could find that had the window I needed in stock. While I was waiting in the lobby for the man to put in the window, I struck up a conversation with the lady behind the front desk. It was an easy conversation, because I could appreciate her job. Her work was similar to mine. All day long she had to deal with customers and service guys that waited until they were fifteen miles from the shop before reading a work order, only to learn that they didn't grab everything that they needed. Anyway, we talked for quite awhile. During the conversation, she told me of this new pie shop that just opened next door, and if I liked pie, I really should try it. Well, just then the installer came in and said my van was ready. I paid the bill, thanked the woman for the nice conversation and informed her that if I did decide to stop and get a piece of pie that I would get a piece for her. I went out to the van, jumped in, closed the door, and all the doors immediately LOCKED. Don't you just love it? My beloved wife is jealous.

I dream a lot about Annette. For the most part, they usually take place in the bedroom, and if we're not already undressed, we're getting there. Those dreams, I'm sure, are sparked by my desire for her. There are other dreams, though, that take place in a myriad of different places. These dreams usually come with some sort of message. One dream she came and simply said, "I'm sorry." I'm not sure what she was sorry for, but I guess she needed to say it. Other dreams, we could be walking in the woods, playing cards, or just sitting there. For the most part, they are short in length and deal with one specific topic. My point is, be open to different kinds of visits. In some strange way, I believe she is out there, and she is with all of her friends and family that have gone before her. In one dream my dad showed up and said, "I see her around," and he was laughing like he had just heard a joke and had seen me standing next to him. You never know who will show up.

Firsts, Seconds, Thirds, Fourths . . .

Tammy, our friend from Chicago, lost her sister recently. The boys and I went to the funeral. It was a nice ceremony, and afterward they had a luncheon in the church hall. It hadn't been long since Annette died, and the service brought back a great deal of sorrow. Not being in much of a mood for company, I left the hall and went back into the church to sit quietly. I pulled Annette's picture out of my pocket. With her picture in my hand and a tear in my eye, I sat quietly wondering why. Why did she have to die so young? Why did she have to leave me just as our life together was coming into its prime?

After a while, John came in and sat down, asking if there was anything he could do. John definitely does not understand what I'm going through, but the wonderful thing about John is, he will tell me that he has no idea. And as much as he wants to help, he wants to try and understand.

Anyway, he asked, "Have you had times when you know that something peculiar is going on and that it is Annette trying to tell you that she is with you and that she is OK?"

I said, "Yeah, there have been times."

Then he said, "Well, if you know she is alright, then you should be alright."

I didn't say anything for a moment. Then I looked at him and said, "I wish it was that easy." I know he realized what he said was a very simplistic view of an extremely complicated process, because he just sat there with this look on his face that said, "Boy, I have a big foot."

After he finished the first course of filet of sole, I said, "You know, John. People talk about firsts—the first holiday, the first birthday, or the first anniversary—as if once you have made it through the firsts, then everything is OK. What they don't realize is it takes firsts, seconds, thirds, fourths, and more before it becomes tolerable, and who knows? I'm sure there are things like anniversaries that will always be hard." Then I added, "Do you remember when I handed you that letter that I had written to Annette, and I wanted you to read it at her funeral service?

"Yeah, I remember," John said as he nodded his head.

"How many times did you reread it just so you could get through it without choking up?"

"Probably fifteen times," he said.

"Exactly," I said, "and you were able to do that consecutively. Birthdays, holidays and anniversaries only come once a year. I don't have the luxury of reliving those events consecutively until I can do it without feeling the pain and the sorrow all over again.

I have realized the big firsts that everyone thinks you're going to have the most trouble with are, in fact, easier to handle than the little firsts. Not that anniversaries and birthdays will be a breeze. It's just that you can anticipate those events. They are days on a calendar. You know they are coming, and you have time to mentally prepare for them. It is the little everyday firsts that bring the most pain.

There are a million firsts, things that most people don't even realize, such as the first roll of film that you get developed that is so obviously absent of her picture. The first family photo when you are standing alone. The first time the kids leave for a weekend with friends, and you realize you are home alone. The first time you go grocery shopping and realize that this isn't a temporary duty. The first time you have to go and buy birthday or Christmas gifts that are from you and not us. The first time you go to a movie as a family, and there's no one there for you to cuddle with. The list goes on forever. These are the things that elude most people that have not been where you are. It's not just holidays, birthdays, and anniversaries that are the toughest; it is the everyday things that will never be the same again.

Pick an Emotion

Pain, sorrow, agony, depression, guilt, anxiety, fear, loneliness, anger, insomnia, indulgence, malnutrition, low energy, short temper, confusion, memory loss, and I'm sure there are a few other things going on or things that I went through that I have forgotten about. Grief is not only a mental process, but a physical healing. I know I just mentioned this, but it is very important for you to realize that what you are going through will kick the daylight out of you. You will be down and out before you know what hit you. And, for the most part, you will stand alone, because most people don't understand. No, I take that back. They don't have a clue as to what you are going through. If understanding your situation would get them a ticket onto the last lifeboat of a sinking ship, they would be going down to the bottom. Don't be afraid to tell friends and family members who want to help by taking you to a party or out for a drink that you aren't ready. You will be asked if you are back to work. They are always amazed when you tell them that you're not. I have encountered all sorts of responses including "It must be nice". I have no idea what these people are thinking. They must think grief is some kind of vacation. Run like the wind from these idiots.

There are two scenarios that you will encounter. The first group will back off and check in on occasion. They will be brief in manner, contacting you in many ways such as phone calls, cards & e-mails. These are the people that will be there when you are ready. The second group will do everything they can to FIX you. Don't be afraid to tell these people to hit the road. If they are offended, too bad. If they truly are a friend they will back off and join the first group.

Chapter 6

Do the Work!

You will be told that there are stages that you will go through. That may be, but let me tell you that there is no defined order, and you may even skip one or two. I know I did. I skipped right over the anger stage. Who am I going to be angry with? Should I be angry with Annette for getting ill and dying? Maybe the doctors? While we're at it, let's get mad at the mail lady for delivering the medical bills! Was what happened fair? No, absolutely not. But it is a part of life, and it wasn't anyone's fault. It just stinks.

I've traveled a great distance over the last ten months. The first five months my grieving was suppressed during the day as I focused on caring for Annette and drowned in alcohol at night. The last five have been right there staring me in the face, jabbing and poking every moment of every day. My dad had two sayings; the first one was for the times when things didn't go as planned. He would turn to you and say, "It beats a rap in the nuts." I don't have to tell you how that statement drove itself home when I lost Annette. There isn't a misery on this earth that I wouldn't accept in exchange for having Annette back. The second statement was, "No s---. Eat a banana." This had to do with when somebody became aware of the obvious. What it meant, who knows, but it usually got a chuckle out of people.

After Annette died and John removed the booze from the house, I was left with two choices. I could, as Cindy puts it, "do the work," or I could bury myself with distraction and avoid the pain. In the beginning, I don't know that I consciously chose to deal with the grief by staying away from work. But that's how things laid out. I suppose, in a roundabout way, I chose to deal with the grief by consciously deciding not to deal with anything else. This left me with only one thing to do: deal with the grief.

It has been the most grueling, gut-wrenching, nut-rapping road that I have ever traveled. First, there was depression. Nothing, and I mean nothing, has any value or excitement or joy. I was stripped of all hope; my spirit was beat into the ground and defecated on. I spent day after day in a world of disbelief. Most days, I didn't get out of bed. I was dead tired but couldn't sleep. I was hungry but didn't feel a need to eat. Today, I couldn't tell you how long this lasted. The funny thing about your mind is it has a mechanism that will take all of your most agonizing events and put them away. They are in a place where I can remember going through that phase or event, but I don't remember the details. I guess this is because if you always remembered the details, you would never be able to heal and move on.

As I came out of the depression, I would experience extreme highs that would only result in a crash-and-burn. During the highs, I would be overwhelmed with nervous energy. I cleaned and organized the house, played loud, happy music, and made goals for returning to work. Then I would crash. There wasn't any specific length of time that the high would last. It could last for days, or it would last for an hour. I had one high that lasted for two weeks. I thought I had finally moved out of the grief. Just as I was becoming secure in how I was feeling, I crashed and burned. I fell so far back into depression that I was back at the beginning of my grief. It took three weeks of "doing the work" and counseling before I was able to function again.

I can't say this for everyone, but guilt started to set in about two months into this process. A guilt that, I suppose, is a learned behavior. I felt guilty about not being back to work. What kind of parent am I? I should be demonstrating a good work ethic to my boys. I have the perfect opportunity to show them the importance of focusing on your goals. I felt guilty for abandoning Tom and Rick. They stood behind whatever I had decided to do with respect to taking care of Annette, and I'm repaying them by not returning back to work. My guilt was misleading. What I mean to say is, I thought I was lazy for not returning to work. The fact is, though, I don't know if this is what I want to return to doing. I am experiencing a life-changing event. It is the most devastating thing that could ever happen to a couple. Note, I said couple, because this just didn't happen to me.

155

Annette lost her life because of this, and I think I have it bad. Sorry, off on another tangent. As I was saying, do I want to go back to what I was doing? Can I go back? I was working sixty-five to seventy hours a week. I can't do that and be a single parent. Do I want to continue working where the sole purpose is increasing the bottom line? I view everything in a different light now. What was important before isn't and what wasn't is. I want the rest of my life to mean more than a great portfolio.

I'm still not sure what I want to do. Cindy asked me to please not make any major decisions for the first year. Don't move, don't quit my job, and don't do anything unless I know deep in my heart that it is what I truly want. It has been ten months, and I'm pretty sure that I don't want to return to the same grind I was in before. So I decided to put out feelers and see what is out there. I haven't mentioned it to anyone but Cindy. I don't want to burn any bridges.

There are still things that I'm not ready to do yet. I have tried returning to church a few times, but I get into the first song, and I break down in tears. I'm hesitant about going to the kids' functions at school. I go for them, but I feel that I'm no longer me; I'm the guy that just lost his wife. That makes me very uncomfortable. Family events are getting better, but I can't help but look around and see everyone else with their wives. It's a tough reminder of where I'm at.

I'm void of all feelings or excitement for the opposite sex. We have a lake in our subdivision. I spent many days this summer down there with the boys. Women are everywhere in bathing suits that don't contain enough material to make a sock, and there's nothing. It's almost like I'm living in another world. The sights, the sounds, the fragrances that aroused me before don't exist.

I have this feeling that right now I only exist. I'm not living, I'm not alive. Cindy tells me that it will come back, but at this moment I can't see it.

You will be expected to always be moving forward. Forget it. Grief is a series of ups and downs. Not like a car that is traveling down a road filled with hills and valley's either, because regardless of the height of the hills or the depth of the valley's the car is always moving forward toward the end. You will find that very often, at least in the beginning and middle, that you may fall back a few steps, almost as if your body is saying, "Whoa, Nellie! You're moving too fast." You thought you were rounding second when the umpire ruled it a foul ball, and the next thing you know you're brushing the dirt off and standing back at home plate.

Sleep is very important and one of the hardest things to accomplish. Your body is working around the clock to heal, using every bit of energy it can find. Yet, at the same time, you will feel anxious and restless, which prevents you from going to bed at a reasonable time to get some sleep. And even when you get to bed, you don't sleep well. You will nod on and off, never really getting any rest. Without rest, your body will not have the energy it needs to heal. If you are trying to go to work at this time, you are adding even more stress, because now your body has to share the energy with your conscious self while you try to perform your job. If at all possible, my advice is to stay away from work as long as possible. Don't put your job in jeopardy. If you need the money, or if the company you work for insists that you return to work or you will forfeit your job, then return to work. I would make arrangements, though, to get help around the house, be it cleaning the house, taking care of the kids, grocery shopping, or whatever you need done that will allow you to get some rest. If you recall, when you had the flu or a serious cold and you began to feel better, you would climb out of bed feeling pretty good only to end up back there a couple hours later completely worn out. That's what grieving is like. You think you're ready to resume life as normal and then BAM! It kicks you in the behind.

Be Not Ashamed

If you ask my friends and family, they will tell you that it is my nature to speak my mind. I'm not obnoxious, but I'm not afraid to express my views.

In every society, there are topics that no one seems to want to talk about. They are the unmentionables of conversation. As it is, those things are the very items that I feed on. Those are the things that need to be brought out and placed on the table for discussion. I know that by adding this little paragraph I may upset or even embarrass some friends, family members, and some folks in the community, including some church parish members. In advance, I apologize for any discomfort or embarrassment you may feel or encounter. However, this book is written for adults; it addresses adult issues. Until you walk in the shoes of the select group of individuals that I have found myself a member of by no fault of my own, well, you're just going to have to accept it and deal with it.

I've read three books now on the subject of grieving and skimmed through a couple more, and there seems to be a subject that is taboo—and that is sexual feelings or desires. Whether you and your spouse were physically active or a once-every-three-monther, guess what? You cannot just turn it off. What I have learned from those I have talked to—and, believe me, it's not an easy thing to bring up—is every one of us has had to deal with it. Whether you admit it or not, and this goes for the ladies too, the feelings and urges come to the surface.

You have to keep in mind that this isn't about sex. This isn't about lusting over some picture in a magazine or getting all worked up from a scene in a movie. This is about lying in bed, incapable of sleeping because the pain and grief is relentless. The night is dark and lonely, the house is quiet, the kids aren't banging off the walls. You're alone in that big bed with your thoughts. Chances are, when it does happen, it is sparked by memories. It may be a special time that you recall where you and your spouse shared an intimate night together, or it may just be the need to fill the void. Regardless of the reason, sexual releases are a part of the healing process. It relieves a great deal of stress, stress that you, your kids, coworkers, and friends don't need to deal with. So if you are ashamed or embarrassed, don't be, this is part of the healing process. This is the same as if you were going on a diet. When you first start a diet you are always hungry. Your body is used to receiving a certain amount of nourishment, if you cut off the supply it is going to crave to be fed. It is the same thing with sex. Your body has gotten into a routine based on frequency and the level of passion the two of you shared. If all of sudden you change the schedule, it is going to crave it until you address it. We all have morning routines. Tell me what happens if the phone rings and you get pulled away from that routine for twenty minutes. I'll tell you what happens, you find yourself running to the bathroom because you have interrupted the routine and your body isn't going to tolerate it. It is the same with sexual releases. After all of these years your body has fallen into a routine and it wants its satisfaction.

There are many ways of dealing with this. Some look to a new relationship based solely on fulfilling the need. Others find themselves satisfying the need with loveless one night stands or hiring the job out. And then there are those who deal with the need in the privacy of their own home. However you decide to deal with it is totally up to you. The important thing is that you are dealing with it. Facing these urges is just as important as every other thing you have had to deal with. So give it its do and move on As with the diet after a little while your body will adjust to the new routine and things will be back to normal. Until then whichever way you decide to handle it, know that you are not alone. We have all had to face it and we all have dealt with it in a way that we thought was best. Be safe out there and what ever you decide to do, don't let society idea of what is acceptable and what is not dictate your decision.

Nutrition and Exercise

Out of the bedroom and into the kitchen. (No, not for sex.) Please remember to eat. Try to eat well, not just snack food or fast food either. Your body needs proper nutrition to keep going. If you gain a few pounds, don't worry about it. More likely than not, once you get through this—and you will get through this—you will drop those few extra pounds.

Stay active. If you exercised before your loss, continue to do so. If you didn't, you really should try and set up a small program. It can be as simple as going for a walk. Exercise relieves stress, and it will help lower anxiety levels, which, in turn, will allow you to get to sleep—restful sleep. A good night's sleep will provide more energy for the healing process.

Chapter 7

From Existing to Living

I'm one of those people who loved being married. I need someone around to share my life with . . . that special person that I can confide in and with whom I can share my most intimate thoughts and ideas. I like having the décor and fragrances that a woman brings into the home. I like holding the woman I love in my arms at night or dancing close to her and feeling her soft body under a fine silk dress. The little touches, the details that she brings with her love and caring to the relationship. Most of all, I miss being loved. I miss being the number-one person in someone else's life. You can't get that kind of love from anyone else but a spouse.

This has created quite a dilemma for me. If you recall, I talked about the love and commitment continuing on after death. There is a bit of guilt and a feeling that I am not being loyal to my vows to Annette. It is hard for me to still love Annette yet begin to have feelings or attractions to other women. Though when we knew Annette would not survive her fight with cancer, she made it clear to me that she wanted me to remarry, not just so the boys would have a mother figure in the home, but for my companionship. That was a very difficult and awkward conversation to have, by the way. Regardless, it didn't make the decision any easier. It wasn't until later that I realized that it isn't and won't be a conscious decision. When it happens, and I'm sure it will someday, it will just happen. I will meet someone just as when I met Annette. Out of the blue without any planning, we will meet, and I'll know it is time.

In the meantime, I have found ways of keeping my love for Annette alive. Not in my heart, because she will always be there, but as a part of our everyday lives. The first thing I did was to get a chest that sits at the foot of our bed. In that chest are articles of clothing, cards, letters, gifts, and many other items that I kept. I kept them close so I can pull them out and remember the night she wore that special dress. Or feel her favorite nightwear next to me once again. I also built three shelves and mounted them on the great-room wall. Mounted on the wall just above the largest shelf is a picture of a lighthouse scene that I gave Annette a couple years ago. The shelf itself holds her picture and ashes, along with an additional frame for my picture that I will have taken when I feel I can have a happy smile. Another shelf holds all of her angel figurines, and a poem about angels that a friend of Annette's mother gave us is framed and mounted on the wall above it. The third shelf has a crucifix above it that a good friend of ours gave the boys and me as a remembrance of Annette's faith. On that shelf, I display one of the many Mass cards she received from family and friends. I replace the card on the shelf with a different one every Sunday. These displays may seem a bit extreme to some people, but they have allowed me to accept the fact that Annette is gone from this world. And only from this world—she will always be a part of who I am, who our boys are, and what our life together was all about.

I have been grieving for nine months now. I still have many items left to move into the good bucket, and I still have days where getting out of bed is not an option. Yet, I can see that life is slowly getting better, and although my days are becoming easier, and memories no longer come with agonizing pain, the fear and guilt of losing my love for Annette is gone. I will love her forever, and she will be a part of my soul for all eternity.

Before I let you go, here are suggestions for what you can do to possibly help ease the pain. I did each of these, and it helped.

1. Spray your pillow with a little spritz of her perfume. For the ladies, use his cologne.

2. Get a full-length body pillow; they're about five feet long. Lay it in bed next to you. It will give you something to hug or back up against. This helps remove the loneliness.

3. I use Annette's body wash in the shower instead of my regular soap. I smell like peaches for a couple hours, but who cares? It makes me feel closer to her.

4. Laminate a five-by-seven picture. You can take it with you wherever you go. I set it on the passenger seat in the car and talk to her on long drives. It's also good for taking on trips. It is easy to pack, and you can rest it on the nightstand next to you.

5. Light a candle at home. I keep a candle lit whenever I'm home. (I set it on the stove to reduce the chance of a fire.)

6. As I said earlier, I kept some of her clothing— everything from panties to evening gowns. I take them out from time to time.

7. I will put her pajamas on a pillow and sleep with them next to me. This way, in the middle of the night, when I roll over and put my arm over the pajamas, I won't wake up looking for her.

8. I play a lot of music that reminds me of times we shared. This can be very difficult at times. But it helped me move memories to the good bucket.

9. I wrote this book. Write in a journal.

The Cup Begins To Fill

I thought I was done writing this book. I knew I wasn't done grieving, but I just didn't have anything left to say. Then the most amazing thing happened. After ten months of feeling no emotion, no arousal for the opposite sex, it reappeared in the most unlikely place (that's not the place I'm referring to), which led to the most unforeseen event. I didn't think I would ever again be aroused or interested in another woman, but it has happened, and it has opened another door for me—one that leads to hope and happiness. Let me tell you what happened.

I was at the grocery store. I was pulling into a parking spot when I saw this young woman (I would guess maybe twenty or twenty-one years old, but no older than that) loading groceries in her trunk. She was wearing a pair of jeans—the low-riding hip-hugger style—under which was a pair of underpants. The underpants were not a full panty; they had an elastic waistline with a swatch of material about two inches wide in the center. In fact, they looked more like lingerie bottoms than underpants. Anyway, the panties were exposed above the waistline of her pants about two inches or so. My immediate thought was that this was a little tacky. But then I realized she was a very young mother; she had a two- to three-year old child with her. Maybe that was all that was clean for her to wear or, as was pointed out to me, maybe that was all she had to wear period—so who am I to judge?

Getting back to the main event. As I was getting out of my van, she bent over to get the soda from the bottom rack of her cart. Well the pants went down even farther, exposing most of her behind. It has been months since I had seen a woman's bottom in silk undies, let alone within a few feet of me. I have to tell you, if she would have offered herself to me at that moment, it would have taken every bit of decency I had to refuse. That young woman had sparked a feeling in me that I thought was lost forever. That unassuming act on her part set me onto the next phase of my recovery. Knowing that I could once again be aroused by another woman excited me and brought the feeling of hope back into my life.

Two days later, I went onto the Internet to get directions and the location of a golf course that I was to play with my brother, brother-in-law, and a friend on that Saturday. While on the Net, this woman popped back into my mind, and the fire began to burn. So I thought, what the heck? I'm told that there are all sorts of sites out there that will show me some skin. I've never done this before, but I was certainly aroused by the thought. Not wanting to end up on some FBI pervert list, I attempted to find these pictures by searching "women" instead of "pornography." Well, the search led me not to pornographic pictures but to the personal ads. I took it as a sign from Annette to keep my pants on and approach my newfound feelings in a more appropriate manner.

I could hear the van doors locking again.

I spent the next four hours looking at women and reading their profiles. The important—no, the MOST important—part of all of this is, I did it with Annette's picture sitting there next to the computer facing me, and I'm talking to her about the profiles and faces that are attractive to me. THE GUILT WAS GONE. I knew then that I had turned a major corner in the road to my recovery. I will always love Annette and cherish the time we had, but I know now that I can and will be happy once again. Love is out there waiting; it's just a matter of finding the right person again. I will never be done grieving. For the rest of my life, things will happen. A song will be played, or something will spark a memory, and I will tear up and feel the loss of Annette. But I won't be there alone, because whomever I spend the rest of my life with will be compassionate and understanding. They will be secure enough in our relationship to know that even though I am crying for Annette, it doesn't diminish the love we share.

One Year

Last Monday was one year since Annette died. The month or so prior to that brought back many feelings and emotions that I thought I had passed. When Annette was ill, I knew all of her medications, when she needed to take them, how often, and the reason for taking them. I knew all of her doctors' phone numbers by memory and the names of the receptionists in their offices. I could tell you exactly what she ate or drank, how much, and how often. Then, two days after she died, I couldn't remember a thing. I couldn't name a single drug or recall a phone number. It was gone. I had a total brain dump. It was gone. It was gone until a month ago when it all came flooding back. It came back with all of the emotion and trauma that existed while we were going through it. I was back to not being able to get out of bed. I lost my appetite, I couldn't sleep, and I couldn't turn off the tears. It became so bad my boys were worried. They stopped the sibling feuding, began to ask if there was anything they could do to help around the house, and started hanging around home instead of going to a friend's house to play. It was as if I was thrown right back into the heart of the illness period and the grieving period at the same time. The guilt of looking for a new relationship and the longing for everything to be the same had returned.

The last month leading up to Annette's anniversary has been extremely emotional and tiring. Even though I recognized everything that was happening, I couldn't stop it. I couldn't mask it. The grief just took over; it was in control, so I let it go. I knew there was no sense in fighting it. I allowed myself "mental-health days" when I needed to, and I didn't worry about the little things around the house. I just let it happen.

We're going on two weeks now since Annette's anniversary, and things seem to be getting better. However, I still break down in tears when I stop and think, has this really happened? As strange as it sounds, I hope I never stop crying for Annette. I love her so much.

From the Hand to the Heart

I joined a group called "Young Widowed Friends." It is an offshoot of a group called "Widowed Friends." Essentially, it is a group of people that range in age from twenty-five to fifty. Not that losing a spouse after forty or fifty years of marriage isn't devastating. I'm sure it is. But at forty-three with three boys still at home, there just isn't much there in common with some one who grandchildren are your age.

My friends and I meet about once a month. Mostly we get together for dinner, and occasionally we go on an outing. The purpose of the group is to help get you back into society. It is a place where you can share stories without worrying about killing the mood at the table. What I have learned over this past year and half is, even my closest friends don't always know how to react when I start to talk about Annette. Sometimes they will join right in. Then, other times, they will be lost for what to say, and at that point, they start to console me. I don't want to be consoled; I want to be happy. I talk about Annette and the things we did together, because it makes me happy; it gives me joy. It gives me joy, because I know deep down in my heart I will always have her. I hold her in my heart, and sometimes I feel that gives me more comfort than if I was physically wrapping my arms around her. The love is embracing; even now I have a hard time understanding it let alone explaining it, but it is there and it is real. If you have lost someone that you loved, I hope you can get to this point, because the beautiful part about it is you can do it anywhere any time. You can scream "I LOVE YOU" with the fervor of a lion, or you can whisper it softly in your own mind. Either way, it is just as comforting. When I look at Annette in my mind and tell her that I love her, I can feel her love rush through me like a shot of cherry brandy; the warmth encompasses my soul. I hope we never lose this connection.

One of the most difficult things you have to do after losing a spouse is go through their things. There are those who do it relatively soon, like myself, for whatever the reason. Maybe it is because it is too hard to look at their belongings every day, or because it is a means of processing the grief. Then there are those who take months, even years, before they are able to part with them. I guess I found the interim. I worked my way through Annette's things one by one, stopping often to cry, feeling the pain of our loss. Some days I only made it through two pieces—not two drawers, not two boxes, but two pieces. I gathered different items I wanted to keep and put them aside. Hats, dresses, tops, bathing suits, lingerie, holiday cards even her purse.

One special piece is the nightie that I bought for her. We had planned a trip; we were going on a cruise. I had it all planned out—when, where, and how I was going to give it to her. First, a quiet dinner, followed by slow dancing to soft music in a dimly lit room. Then, back to our room for a true date night. Annette got sick right before we were scheduled to leave. I never gave it to her. I'm not sure why. I guess it just wasn't that important anymore.

WOW! There's that warm feeling again.

Anyway, I bought a chest that currently sits at the end of my bed that holds all of the things that I kept. Most of the rest I gave away to family and friends, and what was left went to the local lighthouse. For those of you who aren't familiar, The Lighthouse is an organization that provides for families that may have had a fire and lost everything or for a mother and children who left an abusive home. One of the things that I learned from talking to those in my group is that the one thing you cannot do is throw any of it out. This leads to a common dilemma: what to do with the underwear and bras. I don't know anyone who will wear secondhand undies. To throw them out, in some strange way, is like throwing out part of Annette, and I could never do that. I think the other part of the dilemma is, those are the only articles of clothing that no one else saw. They were part of that world that is only shared with your spouse. How could I just throw them out? Oddly enough, I'm not the only one in my group with this situation, so what of it! I have a drawer full of panties and bras.

What all of this is leading up to is, from time to time I look through the chest and take out an article of clothing. I sit back and remember that special day that she wore it and then think to myself, Do I really need to keep this? I don't need this material thing. I have Annette in my heart, and that stands second to none. Over time, I have given away a few items here and there. Some I know I will never let go of. However, I can see that as time passes, and the memories reveal themselves and take root in my heart, I will no longer need the cloth to hold.

What's Next

Do you know what's next? Everything. Everything you experienced before you will experience again and again—only this time in small portions. You will be able to process these experiences quicker because, for one thing, you will recognize what is going on. You will know what to do and how to handle them. More important, though, they come in smaller packages. You just moved from the club-warehouse size to the corner grocery store size.

You will experience more of a roller-coaster ride now. No longer will you be set back as you experienced in the early days of depression and grief. Your mood and feelings may go up and down, but in general, they are short in comparison, and eventually, the peaks become higher, and the valleys aren't as deep.

Be cautious, though. Don't be too quick to jump up and take on the world. The peaks can be deceiving. You are at a point now where you can see yourself being happy again. Life starts to have meaning, and you are finding joy in those things that made you what and who you are. I'm talking about personal relationships—work, community and family. Be willing to venture out; just keep in mind you are still grieving. It is at a different level, but your body is still moving the poison out and replacing it with life. The best way to describe it is the way you feel after battling the flu for three or four days. As the fever breaks and your body becomes rested, you get out of bed feeling pretty good. So good that you feel guilty not being back to work. And then it grabs your shorts and gives you a wedgie. All of a sudden, you don't feel so comfortable, and you've lost all of your energy. Back to bed you go.

Take it slow. You've earned it—you did the work if you made it this far. Now it's time to take a vacation and recoup. Keep filling that good bucket. Life is a beautiful thing, and you earned the right to enjoy it. Find love. Share your gifts again with someone else. Think of how happy you were the first time around. Do you think your spouse thanked God for sending you to them? I think so. And, yes, their life ended, but it was you that filled their days with bliss. Hold in your heart that you were the light of someone else's heart. I can't speak for all of you, but I wouldn't change a thing if I had to do it over. The loss of losing Annette was devastating, but the love we shared overpowered the devastation a thousand fold. So, when you're ready, share that light again. Don't be afraid of being a giver of love, and don't be guilty for finding love. If the circumstances were reversed, I have to believe that you would want your spouse to carry on, to find delight and pleasure in the company of another. I know I would, and I know that is what Annette wanted for me.

A Special Thank You

Grief is brutally painful, and I don't know if it's over or if it will raise its ugly head later on down the road, but I think—no, I take that back—I *know* I will be able to handle it. How do I know? I know because I have Cindy.

I was never a big believer in the counseling thing. It seemed every time something happened, we were overwhelmed with counselors and their words of wisdom. Mental health is such an intangible, or at least that's what I thought. I was a firm believer that in some cases, counselors made matters worse. I'm not sure what drove those beliefs; they were just there. I was skeptical about going to see a counselor, but I was in such bad shape, and I feared my boys would fall into a downward spiral and ruin their lives. This is when I agreed to give counseling a try. A friend of Annette's is a hospice nurse, and she recommended Cindy to me. Cindy was our salvation, our lighthouse, in the midst of the storm. As much as the boys complained about going, they always left feeling better. Cindy was there when I needed to cry and when I needed a rational sounding board, holding my hand when I was dredging through the neck-high muck called grief and making sure a safety net was under me as I soared. She allowed me to find my way, pointing me in the right direction and not allowing my healing to stall.

Dear Cindy,

I thank you for saving my life and restoring hope—hope that was nonexistent, hope that seemed lost forever. I can never repay you for your words of wisdom. Your words of support carried me through a time when my world was without light. You were a beacon in the distance that kept calling me, lighting the path toward my recovery. Your dedication gave me a chance to regain my life, to mend what was torn apart. You provided a port for us to dock while we repaired the damaged hull, and today we have set sail and are drawing clear water.

May the angels watch over you and your family.

Love
Rocco & the boys

A note to the couples: if you have gotten anything from reading this book, I hope you can see how precious life is, and the fact that you were able to find someone to share it with is the greatest gift you could receive. Please don't blow it. Don't take it for granted. Find what makes your spouse happy, and do your best to make it come true.

Thank you for reading my book.

If you are grieving, hang in there.

I wish you well. May your life be full of joy and happiness.

Remember, never "goodbye." Always, "see you later."

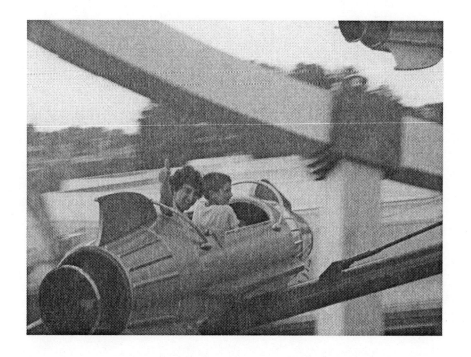

Rocco Ciaramella

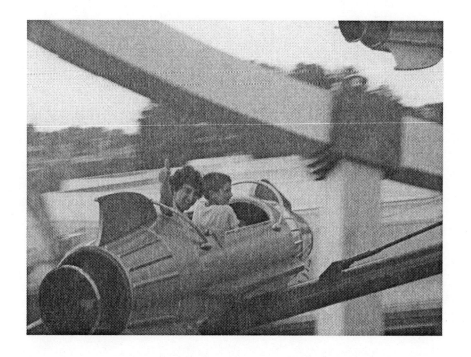

Hey Honey, I'll save you a spot in line

See you later
Love
Annette

174

Printed in the United States
30643LVS00004B/472